The Alzheimer's Caregiver
Strategies for Support

The Alzheimer's Caregiver

Strategies for Support

Edited by

KATHLEEN O'CONNOR

and

JOYCE PROTHERO

University of Washington Press

Seattle and London

A publication of the Institute on Aging, University of Washington. Developed in part by the Pacific Northwest Long-Term Care Center, with funding from the Administration on Aging, Grant #90-AT-2125/05.

Library of Congress Cataloging-in-Publication Data

A publication of the Institute on Aging, University of Washington.

The Alzheimer's caregiver.

   Includes bibliographies and index.
   1. Alzheimer's disease--Patients--Rehabilitation.
2. Alzheimer's disease--Patients--Family relation-
ships. 3. Alzheimer's disease--Patients--Home care.
I. O'Connor, Kathleen, 1944-   II. Prothero, Joyce.
[DNLM: 1. Alzheimer's Disease. WM 220 A4768]
RC523.A384   1987   618.97'83   85-40979
ISBN 0-295-96385-9
ISBN 0-295-96346-8 (pbk.)

Contents

List of Contributors

Introduction

Kathleen O'Connor

Alzheimer's disease afflicts nearly two million people in the United States. It is an irreversible and progressive disease. Its cause is not fully understood, and currently no cure is known. Its impact, however, is widely felt by physicians, families, churches, community home health-care agencies, friends, and the many social and service delivery agencies that work with families.

This volume is an effort to focus on Alzheimer's disease; to present what is known scientifically about the disease and to delineate methods of diagnosing and assessing the impairments of those who are afflicted. As will be seen, the disease originally was defined as a disease affecting only individuals under age sixty-five. At that time, those with similar conditions over age sixty-five were simply considered senile. As it became recognized that senility is not a normal part of aging, Alzheimer's disease has been reexamined. Many conditions that had once been thought to be senility are now known to be Alzheimer's disease, an organic disease of the brain.

Now that Alzheimer's disease has become better understood, however, many individuals think that if they forget a name or misplace their keys they have Alzheimer's disease. There often appears to be as much certainty now that any forgetfulness represents the early stage of Alzheimer's as there was the conviction that senility was a normal part of aging. The first part of this volume, then, is intended to clarify what Alzheimer's disease is and to analyze how to differentiate its symptoms from other symptoms and conditions.

The chapters on diagnosing and assessing the disease clearly indicate the types of examinations that should be conducted to rule out other causes and to avoid jumping to possibly erroneous conclusions. Poor hearing can cause someone to not fully understand what is being said and therefore seem confused. In other cases, a series of mini-strokes can render someone confused and disoriented almost overnight. But, if the change occurs overnight, then the person probably does not have Alzheimer's disease. In other words, individuals may show some symptoms of Alzheimer's disease when, in fact, they have other conditions.

It has often been said that there are two victims of Alzheimer's disease: the patient and the caregiver. Because of the progressive and complete deterioration of the patient, that person becomes totally dependent upon others for care. The caregiver must assume total responsibility for the patient, often to the exclusion of what had been a normal life. The disorientation that Alzheimer's patients experience means that they cannot be left alone: they may wander away and become lost; they cannot find their own way home if they are lost nor can they remember their address or phone number. Many patients cannot sleep well; they may be awake much of the night. Their sleep patterns are erratic. The isolation and exhaustion of the caregiver can be a profoundly depressing and lonely experience.

While the first part of this book addresses the nature of the disease and the ways to diagnose it as accurately as possible, the second section of the book focuses on the partner in the process: the caregiver. It is the caregiver who must solve the problems of daily living, must address the legal and financial issues facing the family. There is hardly any aspect of a caregiver's life that is not touched by the nature of Alzheimer's disease: from joint checking accounts, community property, and financing of care, to daily routines and the continuous grieving at seeing the loved person die before the body dies.

Gaining access to appropriate services is often difficult in the United States. The chapter on the fragmented family and fragmented service-delivery system is but a brief introduction to some of the issues families face. Since laws vary so much from state to state and change frequently, this chapter touches on the important issues that need to be explored in depth by individuals in their given state and according to their different circumstances. The chapter on legal and financial issues can only raise "generic" issues. It does not and cannot give specific answers.

The one common thread in providing care for the Alzheimer's patient is the caregiver who remains with the patient and experiences directly the changing behavior, deteriorating memory, and declining physical abilities. To continue in this day-to-day activity, the caregiver needs support. The majority of the book, therefore, is devoted to the needs of the caregiver, outlining specifically the kinds of support the caregiver needs.

Support groups have been demonstrated to be one of the most effective ways of assisting the caregiver. These groups provide an opportunity not only for the caregivers to find reinforcement for their efforts, but also for them to learn to solve the daily practical problems of caregiving from others who face or have faced similar situations. Different methods of communicating, for example, may solve a problem of understanding. A patient may ask the same question endlessly, even though it has been verbally answered repeatedly. Some care-givers have found that if they write a note, the patient can comprehend the answer. Others find writing a note to be of no help at all, but leaving a recording works well. It is these day-to-day practical suggestions that emerge in the support group.

The support groups' meetings may be most importantly places where people can share their feelings of anger, grief, isolation, and sorrow. Since the group is composed of others in similar situations, the members understand the frustrations and can give the encouragement and emotional sustenance to continue from day to day. Often the support group is the only place where caregivers find support and emotional validation for their experiences and feelings.

This volume is the work of many dedicated people. Many of the individuals who wrote or participated in the writing of these chapters were pioneers in the effort to start support groups, not only in their own communities but in the nation as well. While the case histories and advice are from the state of Washington, the experiences are universal. They are as applicable in New York City as they are in rural areas where individuals and families are separated by great distances.

We have tried to focus on the common elements, the frustrations and the joys. Help and hope are possible. The caregiver need not be alone.

1

The Nature of Alzheimer's Disease

The Nature of Alzheimer's Disease
Scientific Perspectives

Thomas H. Lampe, M.D.

Alzheimer's disease, the most common cause of severe mental deterioration (dementia) in later life, may represent the fourth or fifth leading overall cause of death in adults. Because the risk of developing Alzheimer's disease increases with advancing age, and because life expectancy continues to increase, an approaching epidemic of Alzheimer's disease has been recognized. Up to two million Americans may currently be affected (Terry and Katzman 1983). Because of the total mental deterioration produced by Alzheimer's disease, it has been called the worst of all diseases (Thomas 1983). Although affected individuals seem to lose awareness of themselves and their surroundings in advanced stages of the illness, the process is heartbreaking and devastating for families and friends who must witness such erosion of the mind and personality of their loved ones.

To understand how Alzheimer's disease has sprung from relative obscurity to its current recognition as perhaps the "disease of the century" (Thomas 1983) in the span of only ten to fifteen years, it is first necessary to understand the more general conditions described as senility and dementia.

The author thanks Carl Tapfer, Linda Cubberley, R.N., M.S., Kathleen O'Connor, M.A., Diane Lampe, and Al Lampe, M.D., for helpful comments

Senility and Dementia

Senility

Senility has traditionally been defined as "mental and physical deterioration with old age." Until the last ten or fifteen years, people, including health professionals, assumed that mental deterioration was an inevitable part of growing older. This notion that senility is an inevitable and usual accompaniment to old age has been so deeply ingrained in the thinking of both physicians and the public that it is still fairly common to hear people describe in a casual and somewhat resigned tone that so-and-so "became senile before he died." In addition, senility was usually not attributed to a specific disease state, although it was widely believed to be caused by impaired blood flow to the brain caused by "hardening of the arteries."

The term "senility" as it has been used over so many years remains vaguely understood and non-specific. Senility means different things to different people and it encompasses a gamut of conditions that interfere with cognition. Cognition refers to all aspects of perceiving, thinking, and remembering. Senility is sometimes used to refer to mild cognitive loss occurring in old age, while at other times it is used nonspecifically to describe a severe degenerative brain disease such as Alzheimer's disease. Other common labels that have been applied for many years to cases of senility are "organic brain syndrome" or "chronic brain syndrome." These, too, are nonspecific terms and are used to describe a whole variety of conditions.

Some of the best news stemming from the medical research in the past twenty years on the causes of senility is that senility is not an inevitable function of advancing age, and that when severe "senility" occurs, it is due to a specific disease or diseases.

In order to understand how medical science has slowly focused research into some of the causes of senility, it is important to shift attention to a related and definable concept, "dementia," which is a syndrome that may be caused by different diseases, Alzheimer's disease among them.

Dementia

Dementia may be defined as as an acquired loss of memory and other intellectual functions caused by structural brain damage. The loss must be severe enough to impair social or occupational functioning. Dementia can have many specific causes. However, it is acquired, in that the person experienced normal intelligence and brain function prior to the onset of the dementing process. The risk of developing dementia increases with age. The clinically significant and severe forms of what was once nonspecifically labeled "senility," therefore, are more appropriately referred to as dementia. Because dementia involves structural brain damage, that is, damage to brain cells, it is generally considered to be irreversible.

Dementias are thought to be of two major types: static and progressive. Static dementias are caused by such specifics as head trauma, successfully treated brain tumors, and nonrecurring strokes. With some static dementias there may even be some gradual and modest return of brain function over time if the causative condition can be treated and/or controlled. In contrast to the static dementias, there are a number of progressive dementias that result in increasing deterioration of cognitive ability over time and ultimately lead to an extensive and severe impairment of all intellectual functions. More than fifty specific causes of dementia have thus far been identified (Haase 1977).

Extensive scientific studies, conducted in England and reported initially in the late 1960s, were among the first to identify convincingly the major causes of dementia in a typical adult population (Tomlinson et al. 1970). The investigators began their study by performing careful assessments of the intellectual functioning of a large number of middle-aged and elderly people. Over a number of years, the investigators monitored those individuals and periodically tested them. Some individuals in the study showed clinical features of dementia, and some of these dementias were progressive. When the individuals in the study died, autopsies were performed and included the neuropathologic examination of brain tissue under a microscope. Neuropathology is that area of medicine that identifies structural changes in the tissues of the nervous system and brain that represent manifestations of specific disease processes. An autopsy, the examination of body tissues after death, is thus necessary for neuropathologic examination of brain tissue. Using this method, the investigators were able to describe the microscopic neuropathologic changes that were present in the brains of the individuals with dementia.

These investigators--Tomlinson, Blessed, Roth, and their colleagues--made two important and striking discoveries: first, that dementia was not commonly associated with "hardening of the arteries," or strokes, or other evidence of impaired blood flow to the brain; and, second, that by far the most common neuropathologic findings in the cases of dementia were the microscopic brain changes (plaques and tangles) previously reported in a neurological condition that was then considered to be quite rare--Alzheimer's disease. In these British studies, microscopic changes associated with Alzheimer's disease were identified in 50 percent of the patients with significant dementia.

These studies have had a profound influence on our understanding of dementia. They disproved the theory that most dementia was caused by "hardening of the arteries," while at the same time, they thrust Alzheimer's disease from relative obscurity to a position of still increasing importance. Most cases (50-60%) of what was once called "senility" are now recognized as a Dementia of the Alzheimer's Type (Alzheimer's disease). Other relatively common causes of dementia include single or multiple strokes; mixed causes, such as Alzheimer's disease with strokes; and alcohol-induced dementia.

Alzheimer's Disease: The First Case

The first case of Alzheimer's disease was reported in 1906 by Dr. Alois Alzheimer, a German neurologist.   In his scientific presentation, Alzheimer described the course of illness and neuropathological findings in a relatively young woman he had treated.   This woman, fifty-one years old when Alzheimer started treating her, was experiencing psychiatric and behavorial problems, in particular a persistent and untrue belief that her husband was unfaithful to her. Her disease quickly progressed, and she experienced memory problems and increasing language difficulties.   Ultimately, she became unable to write, speak, or communicate at all, and developed profound intellectual deficits, incontinence and seizures. This woman died at age fifty-six in an advanced state of brain failure.

Because of such severe symptoms of "senility" occurring at such a young age, Dr. Alzheimer suspected that he was observing a disease not previously reported.   He performed a meticulous neuropathologic examination following the death of his patient.   Using appropriate tissue staining techniques, he was able to identify brain-cell abnormalities (plaques and tangles) under the microscope.   Following this initial report, other researchers also began reporting the same specific neuropathologic findings in "presenile," or early onset, cases of dementia.   It was proposed that this condition, presenile dementia with plaques and tangles in the brain, be called Alzheimer's disease.   In 1910, another neuropathologist identified a third microscopic characteristic, granulovacuolar degeneration of the hippocampal cells, in cases of Alzheimer's disease.

Current Concepts

Definitions

It is particularly important to note that until the mid-1970s, the term "Alzheimer's disease," as most frequently used, referred to a dementing disease beginning in individuals before age sixty-five, i.e., presenile onset.   Dementia occurring in such young people remains relatively rare.   As discussed above, because neuropathology of the type associated with Alzheimer's disease is identified in 50 to 60 percent of the dementias occurring after age sixty-five, the historical assumption that Alzheimer's disease should refer only to dementias in persons under age sixty-five has been increasingly challenged.

Current usage of the term "Alzheimer's disease" remains confusing.   Many researchers now use "Alzheimer's disease" to define a progressive dementia: (1) without other known causes such as strokes; and (2) with neuropathologic plaques and tangles regardless of age at onset.   I feel this usage is appropriate. In deference to the original designation of Alzheimer's disease as only a "presenile" condition, some researchers continue to refer to the same clinical condition with the same neuropathologic findings developing in persons after age sixty-five as a Senile Dementia of the Alzheimer's Type (SDAT) (Terry and Katzman 1983). In this context, "senile" refers to disease developing after age sixty-five.

Much debate centers around whether Alzheimer's disease occurring before age sixty-five differs significantly from the same disease occurring after age sixty-five. Some studies have reported that Alzheimer's disease occurring in a younger person is more severe and involves more extensive biochemical abnormalities (Bondareff 1983; Bird et al. 1983). Involved in this debate is the question of whether Alzheimer's disease is a specific disease, or whether it instead represents a syndrome or a heterogeneous disorder with more than one specific cause. This issue has yet to be resolved.

Diagnosis: Clinical Features

The diagnosis of Alzheimer's disease depends both on clinical features of progressive dementia in the absence of other known causes and also on characteristic neuropathological findings. In any clinical assessment of Alzheimer's disease, it is important to realize that clinical findings and diagnostic tests alone are not sufficient to diagnose Alzheimer's disease with certainty. The definitive diagnosis is a clinicopathologic one and requires an autopsy for examination of brain tissue (Terry and Katzman 1983).

Because the initial symptoms of the disease are often subtle, the clinical diagnosis of Alzheimer's disease in its early stages is particularly difficult. Therefore, a thorough medical history and a physical examination by a physician experienced in the differential diagnosis of dementia are the most important factors in the clinical diagnosis of Alzheimer's disease (Larson et al. 1984). In addition, just as individuals vary, the manifestations of the disease will also vary from one individual to another. However, when a group of caregivers for Alzheimer's patients talk about the disease, certain characteristics or commonalities emerge in terms of clinical symptoms. In advanced stages of the illness, more consistent clinical findings develop. Some of the more common features are as follows:

Memory impairment. This hallmark of the disease is almost always one of the earliest symptoms noted. Anecdotes told in retrospect by caregivers illustrate this problem. For example, one victim, in playing bridge, had progressive difficulty remembering trump. Individuals exhibit increasing disorientation on vacation or when not in familiar surroundings. Mismanagement of the checkbook and finances are frequently noted lapses. Forgotten business appointments or worsening job performance for people who have technical res- ponsibilities may also be indicators that something is wrong. Workers have been discharged from their employment for unsatisfactory performance without anyone suspecting that there could be an organic reason for their dysfunction. Typically, memory impairment is progressive, usually first affecting recent memory, the ability to retain new infor- mation. Older or long-term memories are initially retained. Often the memory problems develop insidiously over months or years before medical evaluation is sought.

Aphasia and apraxia. Aphasia refers to the impairment of language. In the early stages of Alzheimer's disease, aphasia may not be apparent or may be just a speech hesitancy, some difficulty in finding the right word, or using a wrong word at times. Difficulty in naming objects (anomia) typically develops. This language impairment usually progresses with speech diminishing until the victim is able to communicate minimally, if at all. Apraxia is the impairment of the ability to perform purposeful motor tasks. Difficulty with complex tasks such as dancing or swimming may be the first manifestation. Many Alzheimer's disease victims eventually develop a dressing apraxia; they become confused about how to put on a shirt or how to tie shoes. Apraxia is also progressive and ultimately renders the victim bedridden and unable to perform any purposeful movements (such as scratching one's forehead or ear).

Personality changes. Changes in personality characteristics are relatively common clinical accompaniments of Alzheimer's disease. They can take a number of forms. Some people become more and more withdrawn, socially reticent, and embarrassed about their deficiencies. They do not interact as frequently with friends, a profound change for someone who was formerly outgoing. As the confusion increases and problem-solving abilities decrease, some Alzheimer's patients can become subject to severe stress. They reach their limits quickly and develop problems coping even with low levels of frustration. This stress in turn can lead to uncharacteristically intense reactions and loss of control, which are manifestations of their frustration and overload. Such "catastrophic" reactions are not, however, an inevitable part of Alzheimer's disease.

Progression of symptoms. Another very important distinguishing characteristic of Alzheimer's disease, which serves to confirm its clinical diagnosis, is the progression of symptoms. It is by definition a progressive disorder. Repetition of cognitive tests over time are helpful in documenting the progressive decline of abilities. A simple useful screening test used for this purpose is the Mini Mental State Examination (MMSE) (Folstein et al. 1975). As the disease progresses, virtually every intellectual or mental sphere of the victim is ultimately affected. With progression, associated problems such as physical restlessness, pacing, wandering, and insomnia may occur. Perseverative or repetitive behaviors, such as twisting buttons, repeating the same word, or repetitive yelling, may also develop.

In the advanced stages of illness, the clinical features reflect the extensive brain deterioration that has occurred. The Alzheimer's victim eventually becomes nonverbal, nonambulatory, and unable to perform any of the normal activities of daily living, such as dressing or eating. The stiffening of muscles (rigidity) often occurs in advanced

Alzheimer's disease resulting in flexion of the
head and extremities in a manner resembling the
fetal position. Also, swallowing becomes impaired
which leads to increased choking. This, in turn,
predisposes patients to recurrent pneumonia, the
most common immediate cause of death in an advanced
Alzheimer's patient. In the advanced stages, some
patients develop seizures or muscle (myoclonic)
jerks. Patients with advanced illness may live
months to several years unable to walk, unable to
speak, incontinent of bladder and bowel function,
and totally dependent upon others for all aspects
of their daily care. The total duration of symptoms from onset to death in Alzheimer's disease is
not well characterized and depends on such factors
as the age and the health status of the victims.
In our experience at American Lake, the average
duration of illness has been approximately nine
years. There is considerable individual variability.

Diagnosis: Neuropathological Characteristics

As mentioned earlier, there are three microscopic
neuropathologic findings in Alzheimer's disease
victims: neurofibrillary tangles, neuritic
plaques, and granulovacuolar changes in certain
cells. The presence of these abnormalities in
sufficient quantity in the brain of a person who
had progressive dementia without other known cause
constitutes a definite diagnosis of Alzheimer's
disease.

Neurofibrillary tangles. Neurofibrillary tangles occur within brain cells and may represent an
abnormality of some normal components (neuro-
filaments) of the cell. Their cause is unknown.
They may be triggered by some disease process that
causes an abnormal fiber to be made within the cell
and that consequently prevents cell functioning.

Neuritic plaques. Senile or neuritic plaques
are thought to consist of a central core of
amyloid, a protein-like material. Neuritic plaques

are usually quite extensive in Alzheimer's patients. Though there has been speculation that plaques may represent the breakdown residue of brain cells, this assumption is challenged and the cause of the plaques is also unknown.

Granulovacuolar changes. Granulovacuolar changes represent abnormalities in the cell bodies of brain cells in the hippocampus. The hippocampus is an area of the brain known to be very important for memory functioning. The cause of these granulovacuolar changes is not currently known.

Diagnosis: Biochemical Changes

One of the major breakthroughs to date in advancing an understanding of Alzheimer's disease came in 1976, when investigators discovered a major biochemical deficit in patients with the disease (Davies and Maloney 1976). The chemical acetylcholine is deficient or substantially decreased in the brains of Alzheimer's patients, in both presenile and senile forms of the disorder. The amount of decrease in acetylcholine appears to correlate with the extent of memory impairment and neuropathologic abnormalities (i.e., the more plaques and tangles, the less acetylcholine) (Fuld et al. 1982).

Experimental Treatment Efforts

While no successful treatment for Alzheimer's disease is known at this time, experimental treatment of the disease is an area that is being intensively researched. Advances in treating the disease have been slow because there are so few drugs that might work and because of the severe side effects caused when total body acetylcholine activity is increased.

Acetylcholine is known to be important for memory. In normal individuals, drugs that decrease acetylcholine impair their memory; and drugs that increase amounts of acetylcholine, if given in the proper dosage, improve memory (Bartus et al. 1982).

Because decreasing acetylcholine may play a major role in the development of memory problems associated with Alzheimer's disease, experimental treatment has attempted to reverse this process by increasing the amount of brain acetylcholine activity.   Unfortunately, attempts to increase brain acetylcholine can produce serious and potentially fatal side effects.   This is because drugs that might increase acetylcholine activity in the brain also increase acetylcholine in the rest of the body, and the chemical exerts potent influences on the heart, lungs, and digestive system.   There are, therefore, few good drug candidates at the present time to increase brain acetylcholine levels without risking disruption of other body functions. This problem has recently led researchers to try to deliver acetylcholine-like drugs directly to the brain by means of surgically implanted pumps.

No treatment is currently available for Alzheimer's disease. This presents a major problem for the patient, his or her caregiver, and all those close to the patient. Like cancer patients, patients with Alzheimer's disease and their families can be vulnerable to hucksters or naive well-meaning clinicians who propose cures even when these "cures" have no scientific basis.   To date, all treatments are experimental.

The initial experimental treatment approach for Alzheimer's disease used the model developed for Parkinson's disease. In Alzheimer's patients, acetylcholine is deficient; in cases of Parkinson's disease, another brain chemical, dopamine, is deficient.   Patients with Parkinson's disease are given a "building block" or precursor of dopamine, called L-Dopa. If L-Dopa is given to patients with Parkinson's disease, they produce more dopamine. The building block helps the brain produce the chemical, and the production of the chemical helps to reverse the chemical deficit and reduce symptoms of the disease.

Using a similar theory, researchers have given patients with Alzheimer's disease lecithin or choline, which are building blocks of acetylcholine. Lecithin is broken down in the body and converted to choline. Unfortunately, the results of these tests have been very disappointing. It appears that administering the building blocks of acetylcholine by themselves cannot meaningfully reverse the cholinergic deficit in Alzheimer's disease. In fact, some researchers have suggested that the lecithin available in some "over the counter" forms may contain impurities that block choline uptake into the brain.

Another treatment strategy has used physostigmine, a drug that prevents the breakdown of acetylcholine. This means that the acetylcholine that *is* available exerts its effect for a longer period of time. Physostigmine, when given in the proper dosages, helps to improve memory in normal individuals. It has been used in several studies with Alzheimer's patients (Bartus et al. 1982). Virtually every study shows that some Alzheimer's disease patients respond with a slight improvement in memory. Unfortunately, not all patients demonstrate a significant increase in memory. It is important to emphasize that the changes thus far with physostigmine are fairly slight. They are changes that can be determined by having the patient do precise memory tasks, and then comparing results before and after the administration of physostigmine. They are not striking changes, and these patients remain demented and continue to have significant and severe ongoing problems in spite of the physostigmine.

There is an important consideration in treating Alzheimer's patients with physostigmine or related drugs: finding the right drug dose for the individual patient. A dose that is effective with one patient will not necessarily work for another (Davis and Mohs 1982). The studies, therefore, are complicated in terms of determining the right dose for the right patient to improve that patient's memory to its maximum potential.

Intravenous use of physostigmine is very short-acting with potentially serious side effects and therefore is not practical for sustained treatment efforts. The importance of the initial modest success with physostigmine in Alzheimer's disease is that it supports efforts to increase brain acetylcholine and suggests that such efforts are on the track toward discovery of effective treatments.

In working with families with an Alzheimer's disease victim, professional caregivers should be sensitive to the rollercoaster of expectation and disappointment engendered by each new "break-through" for Alzheimer's disease reported by the media. It is best for the physician and other professional caregivers to try to temper family enthusiasm until scientific findings are presented that have been tested. It is wise not to expect too much from preliminary reports.

Risk Factors

A few known risk factors have been identified in the investigation of Alzheimer's disease. The known factors are increasing age, positive family history of Alzheimer's disease, and head trauma.

Increasing age leads to increasing risk. Less than 1 percent of individuals at age sixty-five have Alzheimer's disease. For every year after sixty-five, the incidence increases about a percentage point a year until the ages of eighty to eighty-five. By age eighty, perhaps 15 to 20 percent of those living have developed Alzheimer's disease. After the age of eighty-five to ninety, there is no further increased incidence of the disease. In other words, once an individual lives to age ninety, he or she appears relatively free of the risk of subsequently developing the disorder (Terry and Katzman 1982).

A family history of Alzheimer's disease is another risk factor. The family history issue is a complicated one. Studies indicate that between 20 and 30 percent of all Alzheimer's patients have a family history of dementia (i.e., one blood relative who developed dementia) (Heston et al. 1981; Heyman et al. 1983). While this incidence does not in itself constitute Alzheimer's disease as a genetic disorder, it does suggest that family history is a risk factor. Based on current knowledge, the diagnosis of Alzheimer's disease in one or two family members should not warrant undue alarm in remaining family members that they too will develop the disease.

Rare families have been identified in which Alzheimer's disease affects multiple family members (Cook et al. 1979), and in these families it does appear that the disease is inherited. The potential genetic risk seems to be affected by a number of issues, including the age of onset of disease and the number and relationships of affected family members. Families with four or more cases of Alzheimer's disease (with autopsy confirmation in at least one) are very rare, but are important to current research efforts.

Head trauma appears to be a third risk factor for Alzheimer's disease. Two recent studies have compared a large group of Alzheimer's patients and a large control group consisting of normal individuals of the same age and same sex. Extensive case histories were obtained in both groups. These studies have demonstrated that one of the few statistically significant differences between the two groups was a history of head trauma in the Alzheimer's group. Head trauma was defined as a significant blow to the head with loss of consciousness; it often occurred many years prior to the onset of Alzheimer's disease. In the first study, 15 percent of the Alzheimer's group indicated a history of head trauma, whereas the control group reported only 4 percent (Heyman et al. 1984). In the second study the percentages were 26 percent and 5 percent, respectively (Mortimer et al. 1985). Such studies do not in any way demonstrate that head trauma causes Alzheimer's disease. They report an association, and the nature of the association of head trauma and Alzheimer's disease is not yet clear.

Other theories of causation or risk. Several theories as to the cause of Alzheimer's disease have been proposed (Wurtman 1985). One theory is that Alzheimer's disease is a genetic disorder. Another theory is that it is caused by a toxic agent such as aluminum. Some studies showed that Alzheimer's patients had a relatively high concentration of aluminum in their brains, thus aluminum was thought to be one possible factor in the cause of the disease. Subsequent studies, however, have not supported a causal relationship between the disease and aluminum.

Another hypothesis about the possible cause of Alzheimer's disease is that it may be caused by a virus-like agent. This does not mean that it is transmissible or contagious. The disease is not transmissible in person-to-person contact. It is not a contagious disease. One intriguing area of research is examining the possible relationship of Alzheimer's disease to a rare form of dementia, Creutzfeldt-Jakob disease, that is caused by a slow virus-like agent termed a prion (pree'on) (Bockman et al. 1985). At present the relationship, if it exists, is unclear.

Conclusion

Some symptoms of Alzheimer's disease can be treated as they arise. Pharmacologic agents can be used to control certain symptoms that patients may display, (e.g., insomnia, restlessness, depression, and agitation). Involvement in support groups, access to respite care, environmental tailoring, psychotherapy, and legal and financial counseling are all important adjuncts to treatment.

It is essential for those working with families to challenge or mitigate attitudes of therapeutic negativism and pessimism. Although the cause is not yet understood, and as of yet there is no curative treatment available, it is possible to address and successfully treat specific symptoms of the disease. In Alzheimer's disease, it is also important to recognize and treat associated illnesses in family members, such as insomnia, stress, and depression. By addressing these specific and potentially treatable components of the illness as it affects the entire family, one can make a valuable contribution.

References Cited

Bartus, R. T.; R. L. Dean; B. Beer; and A. S. Lippa. The cholinergic hypothesis of geriatric memory dysfunction. Science, 1982, 217, 408-17.

Bird, T. D.; B. S. Stranahan; S. M. Sumi; and M. Raskind. Alzheimer's disease: choline acetyltransferase activity in brain tissue from clinical and pathological subgroups. Ann Neurol, 1983, 14, 284-93.

Bockman, J. M.; D. T. Kingsbury; M. P. McKinley; P. E. Bendheim; S. B. Prusiner. Creutzfeldt-Jakob disease prion proteins in human brains. New Engl J Med, 1985, 312, 73-78.

Bondareff, W. On the relationship between age and Alzheimer's disease. Lancet, 1983, 1, 1447.

Cook, R. H.; B. E. Ward; and J. H. Austen. Studies in the aging brain: IV. Familial Alzheimer's disease: Relation to transmissible dementia, aneuploidy, and microtubular defects. Neurology, 1979, 29, 1402-12.

Davis, K. L.,and R. C. Mohs. Enhancement of memory processes in Alzheimer's disease with multiple dose intravenous physostigmine. Am J Psychiatry, 1982, 139, 1421-24.

Davies, P., and A. J. F. Maloney. Selective loss of central cholinergic neurons in Alzheimer's disease. Lancet, 1976, 2, 1403.

Folstein, M.; S. Folstein; and P. J. McHugh. "Mini-mental State," a practical method for grading the cognitive state of patients for the clinician. J Psych Res, 1975, 12, 189-98.

Fuld P.A.; R. Katzman; P. Davies; and R. D. Terry. Intrusions as a sign of Alzheimer dementia: Chemical and pathological verification.   Ann Neurol, 1982, 11, 155-59.

Haase, G. R.   Disease presenting as dementia.   In C. E. Wells, ed., Dementia. 2d ed. Philadelphia: Davis, 1977.

Heston, L. L.; A. R. Mastri; V. E. Anderson; and J. White.   Dementia of the Alzheimers type: Clinical genetics, natural history, and associated conditions.   Arch Gen Psychiatry, 1981, 38, 1085-90.

Heyman, A.; W. E. Wilkinson; B. J. Hurwitz; D. Schmechel; A. H. Sigmon; T. Weinberg; M. J. Helms; and M. Swift. Alzheimer's disease: Genetic aspects and associated clinical disorders. Ann Neurol, 1983, 14, 507-15.

Heyman, A.; W. E. Wilkinson; J. A. Stafford; M. J. Helms; A. H. Sigmon; and T. Weinberg. Alzheimer's disease: A study of epidemiologic aspects. Ann Neurol, 1984, 15, 335-41.

Larson, E. B.; B. V. Reifler; H. J. Featherstone; and D. R. English. Dementia in elderly oupatients: A prospective study.   Ann Intern Med, 184, 100, 417-23.

Mortimer, J. A.; L. R. French; J. T. Hutton; and L. M. Schuman. Head injury as a risk factor for Alzheimer's disease. Neurology, 1985, 35, 264-67.

Terry, R. D., and R. Katzman. Senile dementia of the Alzheimer type. Ann Neurol, 1983, 14, 497-506.

Thomas, L. The problem of dementia. In Late Night Thoughts on Listening to Mahler's Ninth Symphony. New York: Viking Press, 1983.

Tomlinson, B. E.; G. Blessed; and M. Roth. Observations on the brains of demented old people. J Neurol Sci, 1970, 11, 205-42.
Wurtman, R. J. Alzheimer's disease. Sci Am, 1985, 252, 62-66, 71-74.

Diagnosis of Alzheimer's Disease in the Cognitively Impaired Older Adult
Issues and Implications

Laura S. Keller and Linda Teri

Assessment for Alzheimer's disease often begins when older adults complain of their impaired memory and a decrease in ability to manage their life as effectively as they might wish, or when a family member or health professional becomes concerned about these problems in an older person. One must then ask and investigate the following questions:

1. Does impairment actually exist?

2. If it does, what is the specific nature of that impairment?

3. Does the impairment reflect a significant decline from normal functioning, given that person's premorbid history and current age?

4. Does such impairment reflect an organic (i.e., medical) or a functional (i.e., psychiatric) etiology, or some combination of both?

5. Is such impairment reversible?

This chapter is designed to offer the health-care provider and the caregiver an overview of important issues in the assessment of Alzheimer's disease, as well as an appreciation for the questions that need to be answered before appropriate diagnosis, intervention, and planning can be implemented. It is not intended to serve as a diagnostic manual for dealing with cognitively impaired older adults, but as a guide to assessing the issues involved in making an intelligent and informed referral to trained specialists.

Differential Diagnosis of Cognitive Impairment

Cognitive impairment refers to any disturbance of intellectual functioning. This broad category includes within it many different combinations of deficits and different etiologies for these problems, some of them treatable and some not. Before attempting to diagnose a patient's apparent difficulties as being due to a particular pathology, it is important to examine whether impairment really exists. Several factors may contribute to patients appearing cognitively impaired on assessment when actually they are not. Any such influences should be ruled out first. It is then important to evaluate the disturbances that do exist and to evaluate causes or contributing factors.

The Influence of Normal Aging on Cognitive Functioning

Cognitive impairment can only be diagnosed by comparison with normal cognitive functioning. In the case of the older adult, an evaluator's lack of knowledge of the normal aging process may lead him or her to overlook problems or to overpathologize normal changes. Changes most commonly associated with normal aging are: slow reaction times on motor and cognitive tasks and mild declines in the ability to adapt to unfamiliar situations or solve novel or very complex problems. A slight decline in performance on spatial relationship tasks relative to verbal tasks is also common. Normal aging does not affect verbal skills, overall intellectual status, or memory to a significant extent (Botwinick 1981 and 1984; Lezak 1983). In fact, even the mild deficits mentioned above show great individual differences, with some elderly persons showing performance similar to that of much younger people (Zarit and Zarit 1983).

A related explanation for apparent deficits is that older people tend to have much less experience and familiarity with the testing procedures used to assess cognitive functioning, thus appear more impaired in comparison to younger test-wise individuals (Lawton 1979). Both of these issues underscore the importance of using norms based on expected performance for the patient's age and educational background rather than those based on a younger population.

Sensory changes are common in older adults. It is extremely important to evaluate the extent to which vision or hearing problems are interfering with the individual's performance before proceeding with further assessment of cognitive functioning. For example, an apparent development of "paranoid" or withdrawn behavior might be due to the individual's inability to hear what others are saying, and the difficulties resulting from being unable to understand and engage in social conversation.

Irreversible Causes of Cognitive Impairment

Once cognitive difficulties are documented, other questions arise. Cognitive impairments in older adults appear in many forms and can range from mild, transient impairments to the chronic severe deficits seen in organic brain syndromes. In the Diagnostic and Statistical Manual of Mental Disorders (DSM-III, APA 1980), severe cognitive impairments are classified under Organic Mental Disorders. The impaired older person is most likely to be diagnosed under one of the Dementia categories. Dementia is characterized by a sufficiently severe loss of intellectual abilities so as to interfere with the person's social or occupational functioning, demonstration of impaired memory, and at least one of the following: impairment of abstract thinking, impaired judgment, other disturbance of higher cortical functioning, or personality change. Each of these criteria depends on comparison of the person's current behavior with his or her former normal behavior; the apparent impairments must represent a change from the individual's level of functioning before problems were noted.

"Impairment in abstract thinking" is evidenced when patients have trouble processing new or complex information and have difficulty dealing with concepts and ideas as opposed to more concrete situations and tasks. They have problems combining information and extracting important elements from it. For example, the ability to explain how things are similar or different from one another may be impaired, as will the ability to understand proverbs and jokes or to explain abstract concepts.

"Impaired judgment" is reflected in inappropriate or illogical behavior; the individual may also show lessening control over impulse expression. Actions will appear unreasonable and lacking in common sense, such as trying to heat water in a teacup or trying to put pants on over the head.

"Disturbances of higher cortical function" are primarily evident in problems with language, but can include other disturbances as well, such as difficulty carrying out intentional motor activities despite intact sensory and motor functioning (apraxia) or inability to recognize or identify familiar objects and people (agnosia) (APA 1980; Kokmen 1984). Speech may seem slow, vague, and rambling, with the person showing increasing difficulty finding the words to express ideas or to name common objects and familiar people. The individual may use the wrong words in labelling objects or in trying to communicate ideas, making speech difficult for others to understand.

"Personality change" may consist of a marked change in a person's style or an exaggeration of it. If the person was neat, she or he might become careless and impulsive; alternatively, she or he might become even more meticulous and precise, even fussy. If the person was careless and somewhat absentminded, he or she may become cautious and methodical, or conversely, more careless.

Finally, to be diagnosed as demented an individual must not show an alteration in state of consciousness. Patients must not have lost their awareness of the surrounding environment even if they are not fully oriented to details of that environment. Clouding of consciousness or other change in state of awareness is indicative of delirium, which will be discussed later. While delirium may or may not be superimposed on a pre-existing dementia, it very often can be treated, thereby clarifying the symptomatic picture as well as improving the patient's functioning.

The diagnosis of dementia is based on purely cognitive and behavioral criteria. As defined by DSM-III (Table 1), dementia is a broad category that includes global cognitive impairments for

---

Table 1

DSM-III Criteria for Primary Degenerative Dementia

I.   Dementia
    a.   Loss of intellectual abilities of suffi-cient severity to interfere with social or occu-pational functioning.
    b.   Memory impairment
    c.   At least one of the following:
        1) impairment of abstract thinking
        2) impaired judgment
        3) other disturbances of cortical function
        4) personality change
    d.   State of consciousness not clouded
    e.   Either:
        1) evidence from history, physical   exam, or laboratory tests of a specific or organic factor that is judged to be causing the disturbance, or
        2) presumption of an   organic   factor if conditions other than organic mental disorders have been reasonably excluded and if the behavioral change represents cognitive impairment in a variety of areas.

II.   Insidious onset with uniformly progressive deteriorating course.

III.   Exclusion of all other specific causes of dementia by history, physical examination and laboratory tests.

which no specific cause can be determined, as well as those for which a specific organic etiologic factor can be identified. Whether or not the dementia may be reversible and whether its course is remitting, static, or progressive depends on the underlying pathology (APA 1980). Thus, once dementia is identified, the next step must be to search for factors that may be causing it. The following subsections detail some of the most common irreversible dementias. The most common treatable causes of dementia or other serious cognitive impairment in the elderly are addressed later.

Alzheimer's disease. Approximately 50 to 60 percent of the dementias evidenced in persons over the age of sixty-five can be classified as Senile Dementia of the Alzheimer Type (Katzman 1980; Zarit and Zarit 1983). The disease is also referred to as Alzheimer's Disease, Dementia of the Alzheimer's Type, Primary Neuronal Degeneration, and Primary Degenerative Dementia. The last category is the terminology used in DSM-III, which defines the disorder as a uniformly progressive deteriorating dementia of insidious onset for which no specific etiology can be found. At this time, Alzheimer's disease can only be definitively diagnosed at autopsy, when the brain is examined for the presence of characteristic neurofibrillary tangles, senile plaques, and granulovacuolar bodies (Jarvik 1980; Kokmen 1984). Even at autopsy, the extent of misclassification is unclear, as some of the pathological changes also occur in the normally aging brain and in other diseases (Schneck, Reisberg, and Ferris 1982). Although clinical diagnosis cannot be made definitively, the presumptive diagnosis of Alzheimer's disease is used when the cognitive deficits, onset, course, and lack of other identifiable factors are consistent with the description just provided.

Many authors have described the characteristic progression of cognitive and behavioral distur-bances evidenced by the Alzheimer's patient (Kokmen

1984; Mace and Rabins 1981; Lezak 1983; Powell and Courtice 1983; Schneck, Reisberg, and Ferris 1982; Teri, in press). Although there is individual variability in symptom picture, almost always the first noticeable deficit is a failing recent memory. As the disease progresses, memory will become increasingly more impaired: patients will lose important objects, evidence difficulty recalling recent events, and forget unfamiliar and then familiar names and routes. Some patients will develop problems with speech, being unable to find words to communicate effectively, or being unable to comprehend the conversations of others. Eventually, they will evidence increasing difficulty concentrating and tracking their own actions.

In later stages of the disease, the individual may become severely disoriented and will have increasing difficulty with motor coordination and purposeful behavior, becoming unable to carry out intentional actions or, eventually, to perform any activities of daily living and self-care. The patient's inability to remember familiar people or to carry a train of thought from one moment to the next can coexist with such troublesome behaviors as restless pacing and wandering, aggressive or irritable action, withdrawal, repetitive questioning, and expressions of anxiety and fear. Attempts by caregivers to deal with these problems are often complicated by the patient's lack of awareness of the problems and resistance to being helped. Ultimately, the individual may become totally helpless and bedridden, unable to comprehend the outside world or to carry on any activities.

Other irreversible dementias. Although at present differential diagnosis of Alzheimer's disease versus other irreversible deteriorating dementias has only minimal implication for intervention, the diagnosis is still important in predicting course and in allowing for future research on treatment of the different conditions.

The second most common type of irreversible dementia is the Multi-Infarct Dementia, accounting for 10 to 20 percent of dementias in the elderly (Katzman 1980; Zarit and Zarit 1983).

Multi-infarct dementia is a progressive loss of cognitive capacity due to a series of cerebral infarcts (small strokes) in the brain. Although in later stages it may be indistinguishable from Alzheimer's disease, its association with a series of mini-strokes often causes the onset to be more sudden and the course of cognitive functioning to deteriorate in a stepwise manner. There may also be signs of focal disturbance (such as visual or verbal difficulties and left- or right-sided motor disturbances) rather than global deficits, at least in early stages of the disease. Later in the course of successive infarcts, the severity of symptoms may show more fluctuation than is typical of Alzheimer's disease and motor abnormalities reflecting lesions in subcortical structures are more apparent (Lezak 1983). Onset of multi-infarct dementia is also likely to be earlier, between the ages of forty and sixty, whereas Alzheimer's disease most commonly is seen after age sixty-five.

A history of heart attacks, hypertension, diabetes, obesity, and/or vascular disease, increases the possibility that cognitive decline may be attributable to multi-infarct dementia. The cerebrovascular etiology of multi-infarct dementia leaves the possibility that some patients can be aided by treatment of the associated hypertension and/or arteriosclerosis. Since the deficits are caused by a series of small strokes, there is also the hope that rehabilitative training can sometimes restore functioning, a hope that is not realistic for the Alzheimer's patient.

The remaining 20 to 30 percent of dementias seen in the elderly are accounted for by mixed etiologies or rare disorders such as Creutzfeldt-Jakob disease or Pick's disease (Katzman 1980; Zarit and Zarit 1983). Pick's disease is characterized by symptoms so similar to Alzheimer's disease that both are subsumed under the DSM-III heading of Progressive Degenerative Dementia. Although differential diagnosis must often wait until autopsy, the patient suffering from Pick's disease is likely to show personality changes before memory loss. The course of Pick's disease may be slightly longer than Alzheimer's disease, but the ultimate global deterioration of the person is similar (Lezak 1983). Creutzfeldt-Jakob disease is a rare generalized cognitive dysfunction believed to be caused by a slow-acting viral infection. Early symptoms include dizziness, fatigue, and confusion, followed by memory impairment and speech disturbance (Jarvik 1980).

Other sources of chronic deterioration in cognitive functioning include progressive degenerative disorders such as Huntington's disease, the onset of which is usually age forty or fifty. Movement disorders are the primary symptom of this disease, although personality changes and cognitive decline follow. Multiple sclerosis also commonly presents earlier in life and is characterized by a stepwise series of losses of motor control, emotional liability, and eventual deterioration in cognitive functioning. Parkinson's disease is associated with dementia in 40 to 50 percent of those afflicted. Chronic alcoholism can result in irreversible cognitive deterioration, as can severe vitamin deficiencies (Lezak 1983).

The diagnostic process is complicated not only by the variety of possible etiologies accounting for cognitive impairment, but also by their frequent coexistence. Alzheimer's disease and multi-infarct dementia, for example, are not mutually exclusive; they may well exist in the same individual. Similarly, in the following sections dealing with reversible sources of impairment, these should not be viewed simply as alternative diagnostic possibilities; they may be superimposed on an irreversible dementia or may interact with each other to form a complicated symptomatic picture. Thus, as will be addressed later, thorough assessment is imperative to tease out the contributing factors in a particular individual's intellectual problems and to treat as many components as possible.

Reversible or Treatable Sources of Cognitive Impairment

In the space of this chapter, it is impossible to do justice to the multitude of possible influences on cognitive functioning in the geriatric population. However, a few of the most common problems will be considered here. Although this discussion follows our presentation of irreversible forms of intellectual and memory dysfunction, in actual practice it is extremely important to rule out the treatable disorders first, only resorting to a diagnosis such as Alzheimer's disease after all other specific contributors have been eliminated.

Delirium and drug effects. It is vitally important to evaluate the presence of an acutely confused state in a patient both because of the association of delirium with immediate mortality and because of the good prognosis with appropriate treatment (Jarvik 1980). According to DSM-III, a diagnosis of Delirium requires clouding of state of consciousness, disorientation and memory impairment, a recent onset of symptoms and fluctuating course of clinical features, and at least two of the following: perceptual disturbance, including misinterpretations, illusions, or hallucinations; incoherent speech; disturbance of sleep cycle; and increased or decreased psychomotor activity.

Delirium may be seen postoperatively in many elderly patients, with paranoid and hallucinatory symptoms subsiding within a week or so (Zarit and Zarit 1983). Some common causes of confusional states in older adults include traumas such as hospitalization, acute medical illnesses such as infections, renal or cardiac disease, hepatic failure, and toxic drug reactions (Jarvik 1980).

Adverse drug reactions resulting in either delirium or dementia-like symptoms are all too common in geriatric populations. Drugs or alcohol intoxication may result in symptoms of cognitive impairment, with chronic alcohol use also resulting in malnutrition and severe vitamin deficiencies, which in turn can affect cognitive functioning.

Prescribed medications may result in apparent cognitive deficits or in apparent psychiatric conditions such as paranoia or depression. Such reactions may occur if the dosage is too high for a geriatric patient or if the aged person is taking several medications that interact in an adverse manner. Psychotropic, sedative, and hypnotic medications are the most frequent causes of treatable medication-related dementia, but other medications such as antihypertensive agents can also impair functioning (Jarvik 1980; Salzman and Shader 1979). The medication status of the older adult should always be evaluated with an eye to possible dosage and/or the synergistic effects of a combination of different medications. The diagnosis of untreatable cognitive impairment should be deferred until drug effects (both prescribed and non-prescribed) have been thoroughly assessed and, ideally, eliminated.

Delirium and adverse drug reactions may be superimposed on a dementia. Both conditions, however, can be differentiated from dementia alone by the acuteness of onset and the change in the individual's state of consciousness.

Other medical disorders and cerebral lesions. Metabolic, endocrine, and electrolyte disturbances may all contribute to symptoms of dementia. Anemias, disorders of thyroid metabolism, diabetes, and calcium and potassium imbalances are all treatable sources of cognitive dysfunction, as are infections such as tuberculosis and encephalitis. Untreated syphillis can also be the cause of progressive cognitive deterioration (Jarvik 1980; Schneck, Reisberg, and Ferris 1982). Normal pressure hydrocephalus is a reversible condition in which pressure builds up due to obstruction in the flow of cerebrospinal fluid. The onset of this condition is insidious and the symptom picture is characterized by increasing mental debilitation combined with characteristic gait disturbances which occur earlier than would be expected in other dementing conditions (Lezak 1983). More focal symptoms may be observed as a result of subdural hematomas, tumors, head traumas, and strokes, with the affected abilities dependent upon the location of the insult. Focal damage is likely to be evidenced abruptly, and in many cases medical interventions can prevent further damage or even restore some of the lost functioning (Zarit and Zarit 1983).

Depression. Depression can frequently produce behavioral manifestations that are similar to dementia. Severely depressed individuals often appear apathetic, have difficulty concentrating, have slowed motor responses, and may complain of memory loss and confusion (Jarvik 1980, Salzman and Shader 1979). The patient's decreasing ability to interact with family, his or her slowness, apparent inability to carry out normal activities, and diminished self-care skills may be misinterpreted as dementia (Katzman 1980).

The diagnostic criteria in DSM-III for Major Depressive Disorder are: prominent mood disturbance consisting of severe unremitting dysphoria, plus the presence of at least four other symptoms of depression every day for at least two weeks. These symptoms include changes in appetite and weight; sleep disturbance; psychomotor agitation or retardation; loss of interest and pleasure in activities; loss of energy and fatigue; feelings of worthlessness, guilt, or self-blame; slowed thinking or difficulty concentrating; and recurrent thoughts of suicide. If the individual's current symptom picture is not severe enough to warrant this diagnosis but he or she has experienced symptoms characteristic of the syndrome for the past two years or more, a diagnosis of Dysthymic Disorder is given.

In differentiating depression from dementia, it is important to remember that the primary disturbance in dementia is memory loss; in depression, the primary disturbance is dysphoria or disturbed affect. Upon standardized testing, depressed adults fare better than demented adults, despite subjective reports to the contrary (Gallagher and Thompson 1983, Jarvik 1980). Depressed patients are unlikely to show the aphasias, apraxias, and agnosias evidenced in many demented patients, and they do not exhibit the distorted drawings and constructional tasks indicative of organic dysfunction (Lezak 1983).

The onset and course of depression and dementia are different: the cognitive impairment associated with dementia usually develops slowly and insidiously and continues in a progressive downward course, whereas the disturbances associated with depression may develop over the course of a few weeks and may fluctuate with changes in mood (Lezak 1983). Inquiry into whether the cognitive symptoms or the mood disturbance occurred first may also help to clarify the differential diagnosis (Salzman and Shader 1979).

Depression and dementia are not mutually exclusive, however, although until recently most clinicians and authors have referred to them as two mutually exclusive categories. Even DSM-III does not allow a diagnosis of Major Depressive Disorder if the patient meets criteria for Dementia, although there is provision for noting a depressed mood within the Dementia category. The term "pseudodementia" has been used often in the clinical literature to describe depression presenting as cognitive impairment (Salzman and Shader 1979). As Reifler (1982) has pointed out, however, this term is misleading in that it implies that dementia and depression are mutually exclusive. In fact, a recent review of this literature indicated that the two conditions often coexist and that approximately 30 percent of demented patients are also depressed (Teri and Reifler 1986). Since the depressive component of the clinical picture is potentially treatable, it is very important to evaluate the possibility of depression adding to the impairments seen in a demented older adult. A review of the few studies of depression treatment in demented patients indicates that such treatment can significantly improve the affective and functional status of the patient, although the degree of cognitive impairment may remain unchanged (Teri and Reifler 1986).

Other psychiatric conditions and stress reactions. Depression is not the only psychiatric condition which can mimic or coexist with dementia. Severely demented patients can exhibit the agitation, delusions, paranoid ideation and behavior, and hallucinations typical of psychosis in younger individuals. As in the case of depression, it is important to have a professional assess the contribution of a pre-existing or coexisting psychiatric disturbance.

Next to depression, the most common psychiatric symptom seen in older adults is paranoia (Jarvik 1980, Raskind 1982). While paranoid ideation can be a symptom of dementia, it is also widely believed that some elderly persons develop a psychiatric disorder characterized by persecutory delusions without cognitive impairment, a disorder that has been labeled "late paraphrenia" (Mayer-Gross, Slater, and Roth 1969). Although differentiation between this condition and paranoid ideation secondary to cognitive deterioration is important for prognosis, both are generally treated with antipsychotic medication. In the demented patient, simplifying the environment and providing reassurance can also help reduce paranoia which, due to the individual's memory problems and difficulty recognizing people, often takes the form of delusions of theft or fear of "strangers" living in their home (Raskind 1982). Identifying previously undetected or untreated hearing loss can also be quite helpful.

Apparent impairment in the older person's functioning can also be due to other stresses that are likely to remit in time. Bereavement is a particularly common source of stress and depression. Anyone working with an older adult should look for recent losses, not only of a spouse but of friends, a pet, an article of particular sentimental importance, or the loss of family supports such as when a son or daughter moves out of town. Similarly, a major life change such as retirement or relocation can produce depression and anxiety. The impaired mental functioning and feelings of confusion and sadness that can follow such life stresses may clear up completely with reduction of stress over time, or if the individual was already impaired, functioning may at least improve to close to the pre-traumatic level of functioning (Jarvik 1980).

Summary of Issues in Differential Diagnosis

The preceding sections have examined a few of the major alternative hypotheses to be entertained when attempting to assess the cause of apparent cognitive impairment in the older adult. Before classifying an individual as demented, it is important to make sure that all spurious influences on performance have been ruled out, such as vision and hearing problems or unfamiliarity with test-taking requirements. Next, the possibility of a treatable cause for the patient's intellectual decline must be assessed, including any medical problems, drug reactions, delirium, and psychiatric conditions such as depression. Salient points in clarifying the major diagnostic issues discussed in this chapter are:

1. Depression
   a. The patient and/or others complain of dysphoria, withdrawal, decreased functioning

    b.   Onset, duration and course of problem
    c.   Precipitating event
    d.   Degree of impairment
    e.   Nature of problems
2. Dementia
    a.   The patient and/or others complain of the patient's diminished capacity (memory, judgment, thinking)
    b.   Onset, duration and cause of problem
    c.   Precipitating event
3. Normal aging
    a.   Severity and impact on functioning
    b.   Onset and duration of difficulties
4. Bereavement
    a.   Precipitating event
    b.   Duration of symptoms
5. Medication side effects
    a.   Recent change in medication
    b.   Temporal relationship
    c.   Use of digitalis, diuretics (cardiovascular problems), hypnotics and sedatives (sleep problems), hypertensive medications, and anti-depressive and/or anti-anxiety medications

Although distinctions can be made among major diagnostic categories demonstrating symptoms of cognitive impairment, an accurate diagnosis can also be more complicated than the simple assignment to an appropriate classification. Any particular patient's difficulties are often due to multiple causes, such as depression, or a stress reaction superimposed on dementia of both the Alzheimer's and multi-infarct types. Although a progressive dementia such as Alzheimer's disease may not be treatable in itself, it is important to tease out the other factors contributing to current problems in the hope that some of these factors may be treatable. The goal of such extensive assessment is to eliminate any "excess disability" above and beyond what is an inevitable result of the untreatable dementing process.

The next chapter suggests using a variety of different assessments to establish diagnoses and to provide a profile of the individual's current strengths, weaknesses, and resources in many areas of life functioning. The "multimodal" nature of this assessment process allows for intervention in many areas even if an overall diagnosis of Alzheimer's disease rules out treatment of the primary pathological process.

References Cited

American Psychiatric Association (APA). Diagnostic and Statistical Manual of Mental Disorders (DSM-III). 3rd ed.. Washington, D.C.: Author, 1980.

Botwinick, J. Neuropsychology of aging. In S. Filskov and T. Boll, eds., Handbook of Clinical Neuropsychology. New York: Wiley and Sons, 1981.

Botwinick, J. Aging and Behavior. New York: Springer Publishing Company, 1984.

Gallagher, D., and L. W. Thompson. Depression. In P. M. Lewinsohn and L. Teri, eds., Clinical Geropsychology, pp. 7-37. Elmsford, New York: Pergamon, 1983.

Katzman, R. Clinical approach to dementia. Neuro-Ophthalmology Focus, 1980.

Kokmen, E. Dementia, Alzheimer type. Mayo Clinic Proceedings, 1984, 59:35-42.

Jarvik, L. F. Diagnosis of dementia in the elderly: A 1980 perspective. Ann Rev of Gerontology and Geriatrics, vol. 1. New York: Springer Press, 1980.

Lawton, M. P. Clinical geopsychology: Problems and prospects. In Master Lectures on the Psychology of Aging. Washington DC: American Psychological Association, 1979.

Lezak, M. D. Neuropsychological Assessment. 2d ed. New York: Oxford Press, 1983.

Mace, N. L., and P. V. Rabins. The 36-Hour Day: A Family Guide to Caring for Persons with Alzheimer's Disease, Related Dementing Illness and Memory Loss in Later Life. Baltimore: Johns Hopkins University Press, 1981.

Mayer-Gross, E.; E. Slater; and M. Roth. Clinical Psychiatry. 3d ed. London: Bailliere, 1969.

Powell, L. S., and K. Courtice. Alzheimer's Disease: A Guide for Families. Reading, MA: Addison-Wesley, 1983.

Raskind, M. Paranoid syndromes in the elderly. In C. Eisdorfer and W. E. Fann, eds., Psychopharmacology in the Aging Patient, pp. 184-91. New York: Springer, 1982.

Reifler, B. V. Arguments for abandoning the term pseudodementia. Journal of the American Geriatrics Society, 1982, 30:665-68.

Salzman, C., and R. I. Shader. Clinical evaluation of depression in the elderly. In A. Raskin and L. F. Jarvik, eds., Psychiatric Symptoms and Cognitive Loss in the Elderly, pp. 39-72. Washington, D.C.: Hemisphere, 1979.

Schneck, M. K., B. Reisberg, and S. H. Ferris. An overview of current concepts of Alzheimer's disease. American Journal of Psychiatry, 1982, 139:169-73.

Teri, L. Severe cognitive impairments in older adults. Behavior Therapist, 1986, 9:51-54.

Teri, L., and B. V. Reifler. Depression and dementia. In L. Cartensen and B. Edelstein, eds., Handbook of Clinical Gerontology. New York: Pergamon, 1987.

Zarit, S. H., and J. M. Zarit. Cognitive impairment. In P. M. Lewinsohn and L. Teri, eds., Clinical Geropsychology, pp. 38-80. Elmsford, N.Y.: Pergamon, 1983.

Multimodal Assessment of the Cognitively Impaired Older Adult

Linda Teri and Laura S. Keller

In the preceding chapter, the need to delineate separate and/or intertwining conditions of cognitively impaired older adults was presented in order to demonstrate the complexity of diagnosing Alzheimer's disease. This chapter will address the specific kinds of analyses and examinations that could be used when attempting to determine whether or not an individual has Alzheimer's disease.

Even the brief overview of factors potentially contributing to cognitive impairment makes it clear that a thorough assessment must cover many areas of a patient's functioning. Although the assessment strategies suggested by different authors vary in details, there is general agreement that evaluation of the cognitively impaired older person should include a psychiatric and history-gathering interview with the patient and the family or caregivers; functional assessment; social/environmental assessment of the patient's home and work activities, and the living situation; a physical examination and laboratory tests; and neuropsychological testing of cognitive and memory functioning (Kokmen 1984; Lawton 1985; Teri 1986; Zarit and Zarit 1983). The organization of the assessment package that is described below is based on that which is used by the Geriatric and Family Services Clinic at the University of Washington (first described in Reifler and Eisdorfer 1980).

Initial Interview with Patient and Family or Caregivers

Assessment of the cognitively impaired patient should begin with a comprehensive clinical interview to determine the nature, onset, and course of cognitive, social, behavioral, and emotional impairments and the impact these problems have on patient and family functioning. Information provided by friends, neighbors, and other reliable sources can be important in augmenting the information given by the patient and is advisable to obtain whenever feasible. The family or other caregivers are an invaluable source of information regarding the patient's functioning, especially when the patient is so impaired as to be an unreliable informant. Reifler, Cox, and Hanley have pointed out that "the very nature of the mental illnesses seen in older people (dementia, depression, and paranoia) can interfere with their seeking help" (1981:169). They found that the families' ratings of the presence and severity of problems corresponded more closely with the results of a comprehensive clinical evaluation than did the patients' reports. Thus, it is important for the evaluator to elicit information from several sources in order to get as reliable and accurate a picture as possible.

Assessment of the presence, nature, and history of problems. A major function of the initial clinical interview is to provide a general overview of the patient's difficulties, to determine whether impairment exists, to identify the nature of any clinically significant impairments, and to determine the possible origins or causes raised by the symptom picture and history as presented by the patient and caregivers. The initial interview establishes a general idea about the patient's current cognitive functioning and provides guidance for exploring areas in more detail in later assessment phases.

The first step in the interview is to obtain from patient and family detailed information about the types and frequency of problems they have noted, possible preceding conditions and consequences of behavioral difficulties, and specific examples and descriptions of their concerns (Zarit and Zarit 1983). It is often valuable to pay attention to discrepancies between the problems noted by the patient and those noted by the caregivers, as these discrepancies may have diagnostic implications. The demented patient is more likely to minimize or deny difficulties, whereas a depressed patient may be more aware of impairments or even exaggerate them.

While the information provided by patient and family may provide a general framework for understanding the patient's current difficulties, the use of a brief screening instrument to assess the presence of cognitive impairment is advisable whenever dementia is a possibility. Several short questionnaires have been developed to aid the clinician in obtaining a quick assessment of cognitive status, and these have been reviewed elsewhere (Lezak 1984). These tests are designed to tap relatively simple, straightforward, overlearned information so that errors will indicate obvious impairment. A frequently used dementia screening device is the Kahn-Goldfarb Mental Status Questionnaire, which assesses orientation and basic information on ten items (Kahn et al. 1960).

The Mini Mental State Examination (Folstein et al. 1975) is somewhat longer, tapping reading and oral comprehension, writing and drawing ability, and simple mental control as well as memory and orientation. This test is easily included in an initial evaluation, rarely requiring more than ten minutes to administer. A similarly short and simple screening device tapping several areas of functioning is the Brief Cognitive Rating Scale, which consists of the clinician's ratings of the patient's functioning on five axes: concentration, recent memory, past memory, orientation, and functioning and self-care. This scale is not directly administered to the patient but instead is scored by the clinician based on information collected in the interview (Reisberg et al. 1983).

Reisberg and associates have also developed a rating scale for assessing degree of deterioration shown in the demented geriatric patient; the Global Deterioration Scale is similar to the Brief

Cognitive Rating Scale in that it is filled out by the clinician from information collected in the interview rather than being administered directly to the patient (Reisberg et al. 1982). Both devices require information on the patient's functioning outside of the interview situation rather than being exclusively measures of present mental and cognitive status.

Brief measures such as these are very useful in identifying the gross impairment in orientation and basic information seen in relatively advanced dementias and delirium. They do not, on the other hand, adequately assess memory, calculation, comprehension, speech, and constructional abilities. Inclusion of a wider array of cognitive functions makes a test more sensitive to milder impairments, may occasionally point to the possibility of focal versus global disturbances, and provides an overview of the patient's ability.

As mentioned, once it has been determined that the patient is evidencing cognitive and memory impairments of sufficient severity to interfere with daily activities in some way, it is necessary to elicit detailed information concerning onset, duration, and course of the impairments. The diagnosis of dementia requires that current functioning represents a deterioration from premorbid levels; thus, information concerning the patient's past functioning is necessary for comparison purposes.

Acquiring relevant medical history, such as whether the patient has been treated for hypertension, strokes, cardiac problems, or "blackouts," will also aid in guiding subsequent physical evaluation of a possible infarct etiology for impairments. Some researchers have recommended summarizing this type of history information via a system such as the "ischemic score" devised by Hachinski, Lassen, and Marshall (1974) and modified by Eisdorfer, Cohen, and Veith (1981) to measure the likelihood of multi-infarct dementia versus Alzheimer's disease.

Other medical and psychiatric information. While thorough detailed assessment of medical history may be left for the physical examination, other areas that may be addressed in the initial interview include current and past medications and the relationship of medication status to changes in functioning; history of alcohol or drug abuse; history of trauma, particularly involving loss of consciousness; and assessment of family history of memory loss, cardiovascular problems, and psychiatric problems. It is also important to ask about vision and hearing problems and to take note of any apparent impairment of sensory functioning exhibited in the interview.

Finally, in assessing the patient's symptoms it is vital to include assessment of psychiatric problems, both individual symptoms and possible syndromes. It is particularly important to evaluate the possibility of depression accounting for or contributing to the patient's difficulties. The diagnostic criteria provided by DSM-III can be used as an outline for the information to be obtained. In addition, several useful brief measures are available which can aid in assessing the level of depressive symptomatology presented by the patient and his or her caregiver. While most of these measures were originally developed for younger populations, several have been used successfully with geriatric populations (see reviews by Gallagher and Thompson 1983; Radloff and Teri 1986; Lawton 1985). The most appropriate scale may depend largely on the functional capability of the patient being assessed; self-report scales require fairly intact cognitive functioning, whereas scales to be filled out by the interviewer may be used with a wider range of patients.

Currently available instruments for testing include the Zung Self-Rating Depression Scale, a twenty-item scale which asks for the frequency of occurrence of each symptom (Zung 1965), and the Hamilton Rating Scale for Depression, an interviewer rating scale based on data obtained from the patient (Hamilton 1967). Both include somatic (bodily function) items which are elevated in older nondepressed adults as well as in depressed patients (Gallagher et al. 1982). The evaluator must therefore adjust interpretation of scores based on knowledge of the individual's medical problems. Other useful short depression screening devices that are not as vulnerable to somatic distortion and have shown good psychometric properties with older adults include the Beck Depression Inventory (Beck et al. 1961; Gallagher et al. 1982), a self-report scale requiring the patient to chose one of several options for each of twenty-one symptoms assessed; the Center for Epidemiologic Studies Depression Scale (Radloff 1977; Radloff and Teri 1986), a twenty-item scale which includes very few somatic items; and the Geriatric Depression Scale (Brink et al. 1982).

Functional assessment. Another major function of the initial interview is to ascertain the reasons why the family, the caretaker, or, in some cases, the patient, feels an evaluation was warranted at this time. While the principal concerns may be to obtain a definitive diagnosis, treatment for reversible components, and information on the expected course of the patient's difficulties, often there are multiple other concerns which can be addressed if the interviewer elicits this information. While patients with more severe cognitive impairments are likely to have more problems in other areas as well, it is not generally possible to predict which particular problems will be manifested by a given patient at any time. Understanding some of the idiosyncratic behavioral problems, the deficits in daily functioning, or other stresses faced by the family, will help to guide subsequent assessment and assure that the final recommendations address the issues of most importance to the family, as well as provide important information necessary for accurate diagnosis.

Concerns commonly presented by the family will involve not only memory loss and impaired judgment, but also troublesome behaviors exhibited by the patient such as wandering, aggressiveness, restless pacing, irritability, repetitive questioning, withdrawal, and signs of fear or anxiety such as tearfulness and agitation (Teri 1986). Day-to-day functional deficits can be very problematic to patients and families so that assessment should include queries about toileting, dressing, ambulatory ability, bathing, eating, and grooming, as well as more complex tasks and activities such as telephone use, cooking, shopping, housekeeping, medication management, and transportation use (Lawton 1985). The interviewer should attempt to identify the frequency of such activities, the circumstances under which they occur, the results of management strategies already attempted by the family, the degree of danger to the patient represented by certain behaviors, and the amount of stress and burden these behaviors are engendering for caregivers.

Several rating scales and interview schedules have been developed to augment the clinical interview in assessing these areas (see reviews by Teri 1986; Lawton 1985). Most include assessment of several areas including cognitive, affective, and behavioral functioning. The Instru- mental Activities of Daily Living (IADL) scale (Lawton and Brody 1969) is designed to describe activities common to retired older adults, including assessment of basic skills such as feeding, dressing, bathing, and toileting, and more advanced instrumental skills such as doing laundry and shopping. Pfeffer and his associates (1982) developed another scale targeted at the community-residing older adult, which includes more complex behaviors than the IADL. Their Functional Activities Questionnaire yields ratings on the level of independent performance presently exhibited by the patient on ten activities, for example, assembling tax records and making out insurance papers, preparing a balanced meal, remembering appointments and medications, and successfully traveling alone out of the neighborhood. It also allows for rating whether the individual would be capable of performing a certain activity, even if not presently doing so.

The Dementia Rating Scale developed by Blessed, Tomlinson, and Roth (1968) measures "changes in performance of everyday activities" and, as the name implies, it was specifically developed for demented populations. Information obtained from the caregivers is used to decide whether patients are capable of performing such activities as handling small sums of money, performing household tasks, remembering short lists of items when shopping, finding their way about both indoors or outdoors on familiar streets, and being able to recall recent events. A patient's level of impairment in eating, dressing, and toileting is also assessed.

A longer assessment device, the Memory and Behavior Problems Checklist (Zarit, Reever, and Bach-Peterson 1981; Zarit and Zarit 1983) lists twenty-eight common problems associated with dementia and asks the caregiver to rate the frequency with which each behavior occurs. An interesting aspect of this scale is that it also asks the caregivers to rate how much each behavior bothers or upsets them when it does occur. Zarit (1982) found that the cross-product of the frequency with which problems occur and the family's rating of how disturbing the problems are predicts the impact of the patient's illness on the family better than frequency ratings alone.

A number of other assessment scales exist as well (e.g., Haycox 1980; Moore et al. 1982; Greene et al. 1982) and can be helpful in identifying and quantifying the behavioral disturbances evidenced in Alzheimer's disease patients.

Social and Environmental Assessment

Evaluation of the patient's current functioning necessarily involves evaluation of the interaction between the patient and his or her environmental and social context. Although this phase of assessment is played down in much of traditional medical and psychiatric diagnosis, it is vital in understanding and managing the functionally impaired patient and in providing guidance and support to the patient's caregiver. Often, assessment of the patient in the home setting also provides important information relevant to his or her functional capacities. Assessment in the initial interview or in the home setting should include not only what the patient is and is not capable of doing, but also an evaluation of how the patient actually spends time. Discrepancies between capacity and actual functioning provide clues for potential intervention strategies.

A visit to the patient's home, or, when this is not feasible, a thorough discussion of the patient's living situation, provides information about functional capabilities, the physical and social environment in which the patient lives, and the quality of that patient's present interaction with the environment.

Physical environment. Safety of the person's present living situation is often a primary concern. Within the housing situation itself, such features as the presence of firmly anchored handrails on all stairs, or ramps and elevators for less ambulatory individuals are important to note. Addition of handrails along hallways and in the bathroom can significantly reduce the likelihood of a patient falling and sustaining an injury. Also, checking that the patient has a functional smoke alarm, can easily manipulate locks on the doors, and is able to use the telephone are important safety concerns. The cleanliness of the house, especially the kitchen and bathroom, can provide clues to the patient's ability to carry out basic living skills. Basic orientation can be indirectly assessed by checking whether clocks and calendars are up to date, as well as whether the patient keeps current periodicals or newspapers and is able to recall any events reported by these papers. If the patient resides with other individuals, it is important to hear their concerns about the adequacy of the match between the requirements of the living situation and the patient's capacities. While at this time there is no standardized checklist of "liveability dimensions" to be used in assessing a residence (Lawton 1985), items such as those mentioned above are relatively obvious basic features to be evaluated.

Social environment. The wider neighborhood in which the patient resides is important not only in terms of safety, but also for access to social activities and supports. If the patient is afraid to go out of the house, this will obviously impair his or her social functioning. On the other hand, an older person may feel isolated even in a safe neighborhood if there are no other persons in the same age group in the immediate area and if transportation is difficult to arrange. Thus, the availability of social interaction should be assessed, as well as the availability of adequate transportation and such essentials as grocery facilities.

The patient and caregivers should be asked about involvement in solitary and social activities and their current and past interests. When old interests and activities are no longer pursued, it is important to understand whether it is because of a lack of interest, a loss of competency to participate in the activities, a lack of access to the activities, or a lack of knowledge about what is available. Clearly, each of these reasons would have different implications for intervention.

It is also important to assess the quality and breadth of the social support network available to the patient. Evaluation of the support network should include informal community supports such as religious groups, as well as more formal agency offerings such as day treatment programs, again looking at both what is already being utilized and what could potentially be added to the patient's support system. The availability of additional social supports may be critically important in the caregiver's decisions about appropriate living arrangements. The availability of in-home house-keeping or nursing assistance may prolong the time during which a patient can be maintained outside of a retirement home or nursing home.

Assessment of the level of stress impinging on the family or caretaker, as well as the resources that might be available to provide them respite, is vital in planning for the future care of a patient. Many times, identification of community supports to aid in caring for the patient serves to provide respite for the family members as well. Additional resources available to caregivers might include local support groups or, if necessary, counseling for family or individual reactions to the stress of dealing with the demented relative.

Physical Examination and Laboratory Tests

A thorough medical workup is an essential part of assessing the cognitively impaired older person. Inclusion of the appropriate medical and laboratory examinations can rule out or identify specific physical causes for apparent deficits, ensuring that any treatable etiologies are identified. When a patient previously identified as demented shows symptoms of delirium or a sudden worsening of cognitive, affective, or behavioral disturbances, further medical evaluation is warranted (Zarit and Zarit 1983).

Some of the conditions listed earlier which may cause cognitive deterioration if left untreated include nutritional disorders, infections, endocrine disorders, cerebral disease, and toxic conditions such as drug reactions. Inclusion of such laboratory tests as serum enzymes and electrolytes, blood cell counts, chest x-ray, a serological test for syphillis, tests of thyroid function, vitamin B-12 and foliate levels, urinalysis, and an electrocardiogram will aid in ruling out most reversible causes of dementia. Additional tests when specifically indicated might include a spinal tap, an electroencephalogram, and a Computerized Axial Tomography (CAT or CT) scan of the brain (Katzman 1980; Kokmen 1984; Schneck, Reisberg, and Ferris 1982; Zarit and Zarit 1983). The latter can reveal the cortical atrophy characteristic of many demented individuals; however, this indicator is by no means perfect as many normally functioning older patients have some degree of atrophy and a large number of obviously demented individuals have normal CT scans. This scan is useful primarily in ruling out space-occupying lesions or the presence of central nervous system hydrocephalus and occasionally in identifying old infarcts (Kokmen 1984).

In addition to laboratory tests, the medical workup should include an emphasis on sensory and neurological assessment as part of the general physical examination. Correction of vision or hearing problems may improve a patient's functioning markedly. Neurological assessment will give clues as to the focal versus global nature of the patient's impairments as well as possible etiological hypotheses. For example, visual field defects, reflex asymmetries, and muscle weakness on one side of the body all suggest the possibility of stroke(s), particularly when superimposed on a history of hypertension or cardiac arhythmias (Katzman 1980).

Neuropsychological Testing

Formal assessment of intellectual and memory functioning can serve several purposes, all of which warrant its inclusion in a comprehensive assessment package. While a CT scan and other radiologic techniques can provide most of the information necessary to identify a focal neuroanatomic problem, these techniques have not been able to reliably identify the global deterioration found in demented older adults (Lezak 1984). Thus, differential diagnosis of dementia is highly dependent on demonstration of widespread cognitive, memory, and functional impairment through neuropsychological testing. A thorough cognitive evaluation can reveal areas of intact functioning that were masked by the patient's depressed presentation. On the other hand, a superficially well-functioning patient with intact verbal skills may be shown on testing to have severe memory and problem-solving impairments that would interfere with his or her ability to adapt to new situations or to show good judgment in tasks of daily living.

If neuropsychological testing is performed before a more extensive physical evaluation has been completed, results may also suggest etiologic hypotheses to be explored. While techniques such as the CT scan are indicated to definitively establish the presence of focal disturbances, an inconsistent pattern of deficits shown on testing may provide motivation to follow up with more extensive exploration of possible focal deficits with radiographic techniques. Other behavioral observations such as severe concentration problems or scattered deficits seen on testing might clue the evaluator to explore the possibility of alcoholism or other toxic reactions contributing to the patient's impairments. Departures from the pattern expected for the Alzheimer's patient can thus be used to guide exploration of other etiologic hypotheses.

Sometimes the differential diagnosis of what is causing a particular patient's difficulties will depend largely on observation of the course of impairments over time. Neuropsychological testing is extremely useful in this context to provide a standardized measure of the patient's functioning that can be repeated over time for comparison purposes. Such information is necessary to determine whether a progressively deteriorating condition is present, or whether some improvement may be seen, as in certain stroke cases. Repeated testing can also provide a measure of whether medication or other treatment strategies have made any impact on the patient's cognitive functioning. Finally, even when diagnostic issues are not in question, neuropsychological assessment of the patient's mental and functional status can provide a profile of relative strengths and weaknesses that can be used in management planning.

The interpretation of standardized cognitive measures requires the expertise of a psychologist well versed in the test performance to be expected of normal older adults in addition to those suffering from various types of impairments. In many cases, interpretation of tests also depends on the knowledge of how the patient may have scored earlier in life, since impairment can only be diagnosed if it is clear that the individual has deteriorated from premorbid level of functioning. Although premorbid test scores are rarely available, estimations of the patient's premorbid level can be made.

A work group on diagnosis of Alzheimer's disease established by the National Institute of Neurological and Communicative Disorders and Stroke (NINCDS) and the Alzheimer's Disease and Related Disorders Association (ADRDA) recently proposed seven areas of cognition to be evaluated in assessing the presence and degree of dementia. These areas are: orientation, attention, language, memory, purposeful motor movements (praxis), visual perception, problem-solving, and social functioning (McKhann et al. 1984). The last area, social functioning, is usually included in other phases of assessment rather than being evaluated by formal psychometric means. The other areas are included in most cognitive testing batteries recommended for older adults (see reviews by Albert 1981; Fuld 1983; Lezak 1983, 1984).

Neuropsychological assessment can be performed at several levels, depending on the ability of the patient to tolerate testing and the level of detail required by the assessment. We have already named a few of the basic cognitive screening devices, such as the Mental Status Exam and the Mini Mental State Exam, which can be incorporated into the intake interview. These tests provide a general indication of whether the patient is indeed experiencing generalized cognitive impairments. More detail can be provided by a slightly longer examination such as the Dementia Rating Scale (Coblentz et al. 1973), which assesses a wide variety of cognitive functions including attention, initiation and perseverance, conceptualization, memory, and construction.

More extensive evaluation can include a selection of tests chosen to assess given functions in more detail. Orientation is usually assessed through questions concerning personal information such as age, temporal information such as date and chronological sequencing of past events, and awareness of current location. Orientation to person, place, and time is included in virtually all assessments of mental status no matter what their length. Another basic area to be assessed is simple attention. Auditory tasks such as the span of mathematical digits, which requires the patient to immediately recall a string of numbers, provide a quick assessment of the patient's ability to sustain auditory attention. Ability to sustain visual attention might be assessed through a task requiring the patient to read a large array of letters and cancel a certain one with a penciled mark (letter cancellation) or through slightly more complex tasks such as the Trail-Making Test Part A, in which the patient is required to connect numbered circles in sequential order.

Assessment of language is a complex task that requires a variety of different tasks in order to assess both expressive and receptive functions, that is, the ability to express thoughts clearly and to understand verbal information. Areas to be assessed include comprehension of spoken language, reading comprehension, ability to repeat verbal messages and to read aloud, ability to express an idea in writing, fund of vocabulary knowledge, verbal fluency, and ability to name common objects. Patients with Alzheimer's disease usually have increasing difficulty finding the words with which to label people and objects.

The assessment of memory and learning can also be a complex undertaking. Testing should include auditory and visually presented material, verbal and nonverbal responses, and variation in the length of time over which the individual is asked to remember material. For example, immediate memory span might be assessed for auditory material through repeating strings of digits, for visual material through remembering a string of simple pictures, and for auditory nonverbal material through remembering a rhythmic series of tapping sounds (Lezak 1984). Other tasks are specifically designed to test short-term storage of material, long-term storage, and ability to retrieve material once it has been learned. They can also be varied along such dimensions as the familiarity of the material, its organization, or its meaningfulness.

The most commonly used test of memory and simple learning is the Wechsler Memory Scale (WMS, Wechsler 1945), which includes tests of orientation, mental control, immediate recall of logical verbal material, learning of associated word pairs, digit span, and immediate recall of figures. Most evaluators now add a delayed recall procedure to this test to assess longer term retention as well (Russell 1975). The Fuld Object-Memory Evaluation (Fuld 1978) is a newer test that is particularly useful with the demented older adult. It uses simple objects as stimuli to be remembered, employs repeated learning trials with reminders, and assesses the patient's ability to recognize items after delay even if they could not be recalled. The interference procedure employed between learning trials also allows an estimate of verbal fluency.

Assessment of purposeful motor movements (praxis) usually involves tasks requiring the patient to assemble or draw something, either copying from a model or performing in a free-response format (Lezak 1984). For example, a patient might be asked to draw a copy of a figure presented to him or her on a card; in a free-response format, the patient might be given the pieces to a puzzle and be asked to assemble them into a familiar shape. Constructional ability, involving intentional motor coordination, must be differentiated from perceptual skills. When a patient performs poorly on a motor task, it is important to determine whether the problem lies in perception of the stimulus itself or in the ability to match motor movements to the perceived pattern. Simply asking the patient whether the figure or assembled shape looks like the stimulus may help answer this question. Other tests specifically designed to assess visual perceptual functioning may involve matching similar figures to each other.

Assessment of problem-solving ability requires a range of measures tapping higher cognitive processes. Verbal concept formation is one area that can be evaluated through asking a patient to explain proverbs, or to identify similarities or differences between objects or concepts. Nonverbal concept formation may be measured by having the patient point to or sort objects into similar or dissimilar categories. Often measures of concept formation also include assessment of cognitive flexibility, the ability to shift from one concept or approach to a problem to another. Part B of the Trail-Making Test (mentioned earlier), is a simple measure of cognitive flexibility, requiring the subject to connect circles sequentially in alternating number-letter order. Tests of reasoning and judgment may include arithmetic problems or the posing of problem situations to be solved by the individual. Planning ability also comes into this assessment, sometimes through specific test items and sometimes through observation of the patient's approach to problems presented in assessment.

Despite the almost overwhelming variety of specific assessment devices available, most neuro-psychological evaluations employ some variation of one of the few comprehensive standardized batteries available. These batteries are designed to cover a variety of functions and have the advantage of standardized administration procedures and norms. The revised form of the Wechsler Adult Intelligence Scale (WAIS-R, Wechsler 1981), for example, is composed of eleven separate subtests that cover different areas of functioning, such as verbal comprehension, visual-spatial construction, vocabulary knowledge, verbal and nonverbal reasoning, fund of general information, psychomotor coordination, and digit span.

Longer, even more comprehensive evaluations are provided by the Halstead-Indiana Neuropsychological Battery (see Reitan and Davison 1974), and the Luria-Nebraska Neuropsychological Battery (Golden 1981). Except for the relatively intact patient, both of these batteries may be quite exhausting and frustrating for the older adult to complete. Selection of the most relevant tests to cover the important areas of functioning with the least stress on the patient is a high priority in geriatric settings.

The Team Nature of Multimodal Assessment

The comprehensive assessment approach outlined above covers many aspects of the patient's functioning and life situation. Accordingly, it requires considerable expertise over a wide range of areas from the individuals carrying out the evaluation. Most often, a team approach to such an evaluation is helpful, thereby dividing the labor according to the participating professionals'

specialty areas. For example, the initial history
and symptom-gathering interview might best be
conducted by an individual trained in psychiatric
diagnosis, such as a psychologist or psychiatrist.
Much of the social and environmental assessment
might be performed by a social worker. The
physical examination must be conducted by a
physician. Finally, cognitive assessment should be
interpreted by an individual trained in clinical
psychology and neuropsychology. The location of
different phases of the assessment process should
allow the various professionals to easily exchange
information among themselves, and to integrate all
the information into a comprehensive intervention/
management package for the patient and his or her
caregivers. It is important to designate a primary
health care provider who will take responsibility
for implementing these recommendations and clearly
communicate them to the patient and caregivers,
aiding them in arranging followup care. (See
Lewinsohn, Teri, and Hautzinger 1983, for further
discussion of these issues.)

Intervention Implications

Both the preceding chapter and this chapter have
stressed the need to develop a definitive diagnosis
as well as the necessity to assess the various
functional abilities and disabilities of the
impaired individual. The motivation behind diagnostic classification and functional assessment is
the same: to gain a thorough understanding of the
patient. This comprehensive analysis will have
major implications for improving the quality of his
or her life and for promoting as much independence
as possible. This concluding section will provide
a brief discussion of how assessment can aid in
treatment.

As has been stressed, diagnosing a chronic
progressive dementia such as Alzheimer's disease
must only be made after all potentially reversible
contributors are ruled out or treated. Other

diagnostic hypotheses that should be considered
were mentioned, including spurious influences on
performance, transient reactions to life stresses,
normal aging patterns, medical conditions, psychiatric illnesses, and adverse drug reactions. It
was also emphasized that these are not mutually
exclusive categories. The health care provider
should always keep in mind that even the most
severe progressive dementia may have treatable
components. Careful diagnosis will aid in dis-
covering the treatable aspects and reducing the
patient's "excess disability" as much as possible.

The range of treatment options potentially
useful in reducing or eliminating reversible
factors contributing to the condition is almost as
great as the number of these factors themselves.
Accurate diagnosis will guide the choice of appropriate interventions from this wide range of
possibilities. For example, treatment may involve
something as simple as the prescription of glasses
or a hearing aid for the patient whose sensory
deficits present an apparent impairment on cognitive tasks. Medical problems that result in
cognitive deficits may require treatments as
diverse as surgery to remove a tumor, medication to
treat an infection, or vitamins to correct a nutritional imbalance. Medication may also be indicated
to help control psychiatric disorders such as
severe depression or paranoia.

On the other hand, if over-medication or medication interactions are found to be a factor in the
patient's cognitive difficulties, the treatment of
choice is likely to involve reducing or even
discontinuing specific medications. Other forms of
treatment may involve behavioral or environmental
interventions rather than medical treatment, such
as increasing a patient's activities to combat
depression or adding a wheelchair ramp to the front
of a house to make it easier for the patient to get
out and function more independently.

Even if no treatable cause for a patient's
impairments can be found, the establishment of a

final diagnosis of Alzheimer's disease can in itself have therapeutic implications for the family or caregivers. "First, it reassures the family that they have met their responsibility of ruling out reversible causes. Second, it provides an opportunity to discuss the disease. Many people can cope best with the problem if they have such facts at their disposal. Finally, it allows both patient and family to benefit from aspects of the sick role, in which the patient can be seen as having a problem not of his or her own making that entitles both patient and relative to certain services and privileges" (Reifler and Wu 1982: 1055).

Including the caregiving system in the evaluation process is one of the primary strengths of the assessment approach presented here. The patient's quality of life will most often be maximized by providing caregivers the information, options, and support they need in planning for the care of their relative. A major goal is to identify the sources of stress in this system and to reduce them as much as possible. Often intervention with the caregiver designed to give needed respite and a feeling of control over the situation is the most direct way of aiding the patient as well.

In summary, the keys to appropriate treatment of the demented patient are accurate diagnosis and thorough assessment of resources and deficits in cognitive, behavioral, social, and emotional functioning. Intervention efforts can go far beyond treating reversible physical contributors to the patient's impairments. Providing caregivers with information and assistance from support groups and community resources, aiding them in establishing realistic expectations for the patient and themselves, and helping them develop coping techniques matched to the abilities of the patient can be the most effective way to improve quality of life for both patient and caregiver.

References Cited

Albert, M. S. Geriatric neuropsychology. J of Consulting and Clinical Psychology, 1981, 49: 835-50.

Beck, A. T.; C. H. Ward; M. Mendelson; J. E. Mock; and J. Erbaugh. An inventory for measuring depression. Arch of Gen Psych 1961, 4:561-71.

Blessed, F.; B. E. Tomlinson; and M. Roth. The association between quantitative measures of dementia and of senile change in the cerebral gray matter of elderly subjects. Brit J Psych, 1968, 114:797-811.

Brink, T. L.; J. A. Yesavage; O. Lum; P. Heersema; M. Adey; and T. L. Rose. Screening tests for geriatric depression. Clinical Gerontologist, 1982, 1:37-44.

Coblentz, J. M.; S. Mattis; L. H. Zingesser; S. S. Kasoff; H. M. Wisniewski; and R. Katzman. Presenile Dementia. Arch Neurol, 1973, 29:299-308.

Eisdorfer, C.; D. Cohen; and R. Veith. The Psychopathology of Aging: Current Concepts. New York: Scope Publications, 1981.

Folstein, M. F.; S. E. Folstein; and P. R. McHugh. "Mini-mental state:" A practical method for grading the cognitive state of patients for the clinician. J of Psych Research, 1975, 12:189-98.

Fuld, P. A. Psychological testing in the differential diagnosis of the dementias. In R. Katzman, R. D. Terry, and K. L. Bick, eds., Alzheimer's Disease: Senile Dementia and Related Disorders, pp. 185-93. New York: Raven Press, 1978.

Fuld, P. A. Psycometric differentiation of the dementias: An overview. In B. Reisberg, ed., A Textbook of Alzheimer's Disease and Senile Dementia. New York: Free Press, 1983.

Gallagher, D.; G. Niew; and L. Thompson. Reliability of the Beck Depression Inventory with older adults. J. Consulting and Clinical Psych, 1982, 50:152-53.

Gallagher, D., and L. W. Thompson. Depression. In
P. M. Lewinshon and L. Teri, eds. Clinical
Geropsychology, pp. 7-37. Elmsford, New York:
Pergamon, 1983.

Golden, C. J. A standardized version of Luria's
neuropsychological tests. In S. Filskov and T.
J. Boll, eds., Handbook of Clinical Neuropsychology. New York: Wiley-Interscience, 1981.

Greene, J. G.; R. Smith; M. Gardiner; and G. C.
Timbury. Measuring behavioral disturbance of
elderly demented patients in the community and
its effects on relatives: A factor analytic
study. Age and Aging, 1982, 11:121-26.

Hachinski, V.; N. Lassen; and J. Marshall. Multi-
infarct dementia: A cause of mental deterioration in the elderly. Lancet, 1974, 2:207-10.

Hamilton, M. Development of a rating scale for
primary depressive illness. Brit J of Social
and Clinical Psych, 1967, 6:278-96.

Haycox, J. A. A behavioral scale for dementia. In
C. A. Shamoian, ed., Biology and Treatment of
Dementia in the Elderly, pp. 2-13. Washington,
D.C.: Am. Psychiatric Press, 1980.

Kahn, R. L.; A. I. Goldfarb; M. Pollack; and R.
Peck. Brief objective measures for the deter-
mination of mental status in the aged. Amer J
Psychiatry, 1960, 117:326-28.

Katzman, R. Clinical approach to dementia. Neuro-
Ophthalmology Focus, 1980.

Kokmen, E. Dementia, Alzheimer type. Mayo Clinic
Proceedings, 1984, 59:35-42.

Lawton, M. P. Functional assessment. In L. Teri
and P. Lewinsohn, eds., Geropsychological
Assessment and Treatment, pp. 39-85. New York:
Springer Press, 1985.

Lawton, M. P., and E. M. Brody. Assessment of older
people: self-maintaining and instrumental activities of daily living. Gerontologist, 1969,
9:179-88.

Lewishon, P. M.; L. Teri; and M. Hautzinger.
Training clinical psychologists to work with

older adults: A working model. Professional Psych, 1983, 15:187-202.

Lezak, M. D. Neuropsychological Assessment. 2d ed.. New York: Oxford Press, 1983.

Lezak, M. D. Neuropsychological assessment of the elderly. In L. Teri and P. M. Lewinsohn, eds., Assessment and Treatment of Older Adults. New York: Springer, 1984.

McKhann, G., D. Drachman; M. R. Folstein; R. Katzman; D. Price; and E. Stadlan. Clinical diagnosis of Alzheimer's disease: Report of the NINCDS-ADRDA work group. Neurology, 1984, 34:939-44.

Moore, J. T.; J. A. Bobula; T. B. Short; and M. Mischel. A functional dementia scale. J of Family Practice, 1982, 16:499-503.

Pfeffer, R. I., T. T. Kurosaki; C. H. Harrah; J. M. Chance; and S. Filos. Measurement of functional activities in older adults in the community. J of Gerontology, 1982, 37:323-29.

Radloff, L. W. The CES-D scale: A self-report depression scale for research in the general population. Applied Psych Measurement, 1977, 1:385-401.

Radloff, L., and L. Teri. The use of the CES-D Scale with older adults. Clinical Gerontologist, 1986, 5:119-37.

Reifler, B. V.; G. B. Cox; and R. J. Hanley. Problems of mentally ill elderly as perceived by patients, families, and clinicians. Gerontologist, 1981, 21:165-70.

Reifler, B. V., and C. Eisdorfer. A clinic for the impaired elderly and their families. Amer J Psychiatry, 1980, 137:1399-1403.

Reifler, B. V., and S. Wu. Managing families of the demented elderly. J of Family Practice, 1982, 14:1051-56.

Reisberg, B.; S. H. Ferris; M. J. deLeon; and T. Crook. The Global Deterioration Scale (GDS): An instrument for the assessment of primary degenerative dementia (PDD). Amer J Psychiatry, 1982, 139:1136-39.

Reisberg, B.; M. K. Schneck; S. H. Ferris; G. E. Schwartz; and M. J. deLeon. The Brief Cognitive Rating Scale (BCRS): Findings in primary degenerative dementia (PDD). Psychopharmacology Bull, 1983, 19:47-50.

Reitan, R. M., and L. A. Davison. Clinical Neuropsychology: Current Status and Applications. New York: Hemisphere, 1974.

Russell, E. W. A multiple scoring method for the assessment of complex memory functions. J of Consulting and Clinical Psychology, 1975, 43:800-809.

Schneck, M. K.; B. Reisberg; and S. H. Ferris. An overview of current concepts of Alzheimer's disease. Amer J Psychiatry, 1982, 139:169-73.

Teri, L. Severe cognitive impairments in older adults. Behavior Therapist, 1986, 9:51-54..

Wechsler, D. A standardized memory scale for clinical use. J of Psychology, 1945, 19:87-95.

Wechsler, D. WAIS-R Manual. New York: Psychological Corporation, 1981.

Zarit, S. H.; K. E. Reever; and J. Bach-Peterson. Relatives of the impaired elderly: Correlates of feelings of burden. Gerontologist, 1981, 21:158-64.

Zarit, S. H. Predictors of burden and distress for caregivers of senile dementia patients. Ph.D. dissertation, Univ of Southern California, 1982.

Zarit, S. H., and J. M. Zarit. Cognitive impairment. In P. M. Lewinsohn and L. Teri, eds., Clinical Geropsychology, pp. 38-80. Elmsford, N.Y.: Pergamon, 1983.

Zung, W. A self-rating depression scale. Arch Gen Psychiatry, 1965, 12:63-70.

2
The Patient, the Caregiver, and the Family

Supporting the Alzheimer's Caregiver

Judy Gellatly

I. Why the Caregiver Needs Support

All caregivers and care providers, both amateur and
professional, part-time and full-time, need and
must have support. The caregiver's job is a complex
mixture of tasks, problems, and emotions. For the
manager of an Alzheimer's patient, the needs for
support are many and continuing.

An Alzheimer's patient is an intelligent adult
whose brain is malfunctioning. The brain goes
haywire until all learned facts, memories, and
functions are lost. The disease is a trip to
oblivion without any guidebook or timetable. From
the first moment of the first suspicion that
something is wrong with that person's usually
normal behavior, judgment, or memory, to the point
when the patient is forever gone mentally, the time
of institutionalization, and the finality of death,
the patient's caregiver needs support.

This chapter describes the impact of the
disease on the family, the kinds of support that
family caregivers need, and the unique role that
support groups can play in assisting the caregiver
through a most difficult process. There are many
resources available to families who face this
horrible disease. By understanding some of its
impact on the family, agency personnel can help
find the most appropriate ways to assist the
individual and the family. One of the most important supports, however, has been the creation of
support groups that aid the individual in his or
her caregiving efforts.

Impact of the Illness on the Patient and Family

Even before diagnosis, family members closest to
the victim-to-be suspect that something is amiss.

Puzzling changes in usual behavior, poor judgment, and memory loss are noted by anyone close to the person. But many of the changes are small things at first, and can easily be excused or rationalized. Besides, the person in question is just fine most of the time. Then, as his or her personality begins to change, often with sudden mood swings, contradictory statements, illogical reasoning, the observer in the family knows that something is wrong. But what is to be done? Where do families turn? To family members? They may not be helpful and may instead blame advancing age, medications, mid-life crisis, or provocation by the caregiver. If the disease does not worsen right away, there may be a time of denial. The family may conclude that there is really nothing wrong. They may assume blame for what has happened and try to be more considerate and understanding. At this stage, the caregiver is designated by circumstances (the only available person), or by agreement (the family decides who the caregiver will be), and the need for support begins.

After this insidious beginning, the patient begins to show some definitely decreasing abilities, loss of skills, loss of memory, confusion, disorientation. With these symptoms increasing, the caregiver seeks professional help, often the consultation of the family doctor. In some cases a misdiagnosis, such as arteriosclerosis, is made, and medication is prescribed to treat that specific illness. After a brief feeling of relief, however, the caregiver comes to realize that there is little or no change in the problem behaviors and is more baffled than ever. Some get quite a runaround, going from one clinic or physician to another.

Finally, the diagnosis of Alzheimer's disease is made by exclusion. Tests are given to eliminate the possibility of several other treatable diseases that have similar symptoms. The physician explains that it is probably Alzheimer's disease, a case of dementia that is incurable and untreatable. The word "probably" is the best the physician can say, because the physician only knows what the disease is not, and that it is some type of neurological dementia. Only through an autopsy, with the brain tissue examined under a microscope, can one detect the neurofibrillary tangles and plaques that prevent messages from traveling properly through the 3 billion cells in the brain.

The diagnosis might be met by the family and victim with denial, and might send them on yet another round of searches for a different opinion. The diagnosis, damning and hopeless as it is, has a traumatic impact on the victim, the caregiver, and the family. As with many shocks, the "fight or flight," "cope or cop out" response is felt by those nearest to the caregiving situation. The flight response brings more denial, thoughts of divorce, of institutionalizing the victim, or some withdrawal tactics to avoid responsibilities. Some families may follow this route, but more often, the designated caregiver accepts the responsibilities and the coping begins.

Emotional support. The first and continuing need of the caregiver is for emotional support. The caregiver's initial reaction to the patient's off-beat statements, actions, and opinions is emotional. When the patient is angry, the caregiver gets angry. The increasing helplessness of the patient causes frustration. The uncertainties of the patient's behavior beget anxieties about what will be done next. The insults spoken by the victim cause hurt feelings. There may be danger of the patient inflicting physical abuse. Fear is often present, fear for the self, and fear for the patient. Caregiving is an emotional rollercoaster, and the pervading emotion is grief, a never-ending, on-going, increasing grief over the inexorable tragedy of lost intelligence. Such a burden cannot be carried alone.

Information. The second need is education. The caregiver assumes a new and often unaccustomed role. For example, learning about the illness itself is a major need that is seldom satisfied by relying solely on the physician. Information about resources in the community must be gleaned somehow, by someone. Counsel on legal and fiscal matters must be sought. Guidance on management of the disease and planning future caregiving needs are both helpful and necessary. The caregiver must also learn the logistics of patient handling as different situations develop. To acquire all this information, the experience of others is as necessary as reading the available publications.

Psychological understanding. The third need is for psychological understanding. When a normal, sane person is caring for a person with seemingly erratic behavior that is caused by brain failure, that caregiver must become a psychologist. The caregiver must be an observer and analyst of the patient's actions, must learn the techniques of non-verbal communication when the patient can no longer speak, and must be able to take a clinical point of view. The psychological phases of grief need to be discussed, as does the diffusion of anger. These and many more psychological techniques can best be understood through professional counsel in a support group with other caregivers, where role playing and experience sharing can be accomplished with complete confidentiality.

Relationships. The fourth need concerns relationships. Supportive help is needed to delineate the patient-caregiver interaction: when and how to offer help, raise spirits, and withstand setbacks. The family may be divided as to some aspects of the patient's care. The young may be impatient with and obnoxious to the patient. Friends of the caregiver and patient may stop coming by. How can the caregiver relate to the professionals in the case in order to get maximum service? Again, supportive groups can often help find the answers and offer solutions.

Self-care. The great need of caregivers for support can cause them to neglect caring for their own needs. This is very easy to do when a person is dedicated to caring for another. The caregiver's

philosophy is usually, "Non-ministrari sed minis-
trare" (not to be ministered unto, but to minister)
The caregiver will be better able to "minister" to
the patient, however, if that caregiver takes care
of his or her own mental and physical health. In a
support group, he or she can realize the value of
respite time, new friends, shared hobbies, avoiding
feelings of being trapped (cabin fever), and of
martyrdom. Best is the bounce of feedback, the
cheering on of others who appreciate the caregiver's burden.

Philosophical outlook. The sixth need is for
developing a new philosophy of life. The anxieties
and uncertainties of life with an Alzheimer's
patient do sometimes lead to a loss of faith or a
lost, alone feeling and belief that life has no
meaning. Those feelings could lead to depression,
more than just a "blue day." If disillusion is
great, such feelings can and should be talked out
in a friendly and confidential group that can make
encouraging and enspiriting suggestions.

Problems of caregiving. The seventh and continuing need is for logistical or mechanical help
in solving problems of caregivers. Some of these
are getting the patient to go from here to there;
getting him or her to eat; dress or undress; drive
a car; take a walk; bathe; or what not. Problems of
this type can often be solved by others in the
group based on their own trial-and-error experience.

Grieving. The final need is for help and
support in facing the end of the caregiver-patient
relationship, when the caregiver is replaced by
another person, or the patient is put in a nursing
home, and, finally, when the patient dies. The
grieving at death is often complicated by remorse
and guilt, and help is needed in closing that
chapter and surviving the loss. The loneliness of
separation from the patient can be devastating to
the caregiver, again with remorse and guilt often
present.

Advantages of a Support Group

A support group can rally round to help, because many of its members will have worked through this difficult sadness. A great advantage of a support group is the mysterious fact that within a well-led session, the caregiver can speak of the unspeakable, be it a scary problem, a family feud, or a secret (guilty or not). One group member expressed it after exposing a detail of her life: "There it is. Now I can talk about anything, anything at all, and I know I'll get no disapproval, only empathy and help from you all." The needs are so great, the results so gratifying, that the support group is truly a necessity for every Alzheimer caregiver.

Role of Suport Groups: Structure and Activities

Starting a support group requires time and ingenuity; keeping a successful group going requires even more. The first and lasting goal of a support group for Alzheimer's disease caregivers must be the support members give each other. Because of the nature of the illness, from its insidious beginning to its tragic end, caregivers are on an emotional rollercoaster of chores, grief, strained relationships, legal and financial concerns, logistical problems, and the unpredictable and amazing behaviors of the Alzheimer's victim.

The Alzheimer's support group is often an open-ended, participatory type of group, and like a stream-fed lake, is ever-changing. New members join, others drop out or graduate, so that the attendees at most sessions are a mix of neophytes, middlings, and old timers expert at the tasks of caregiving. That mix provides a continual challenge to the leadership to maintain attendance and interest in areas of programming, agendas, and group dynamics. The common denominators are the similarity of burdens and the singleminded focus on the many facets of one subject: Alzheimer's disease. They are shared by caregivers who are spouses, siblings, children, nurses, health care personnel--in fact, anyone who is concerned with a patient.

Because attendance and participation at meetings are voluntary, group leaders must try to ensure that individual needs are being met, and strive to maintain the group as a lively and valuable exper- ience. This will assure the on-going life of the group.

Each person who attends an Alzheimer's support group meeting has probably been a member of some other kind of group: a book club, a church activity, a sports team. However, the experience of a self-help group might be new. The person may not have experience with a group that stresses depth of personal disclosure, therapeutic sharing, and interdependence. The person may be unaccustomed to a group in which everyone participates, in which leaders are facilitators, and in which each member has a responsibility to help others, as well as to help him- or herself. Therefore, the newcomer should be eased into this type of group process, perhaps by just being an observer at first. The group leader can be instrumental in making the new person feel welcome, and in encouraging the on- going members to recall their own feelings of uneasiness when they first joined the group and to help make the new members feel comfortable.

The patients being cared for by group members will be at different stages of the disease, so that the caregivers' specific problems will probably vary tremendously. Newer attendees who might be reluctant to open up their own Pandora's box of troubles and problems, should not be overwhelmed by hearing about problems of later-stage patients. Nor should long-term members be bored with contin- ual explanations of the stages of the disease that they already know or have experienced.

The problem of education about the illness itself is a difficult one for the group leader.

Newcomers say they want to hear all about the disease. Oldtimers have been through all that and they want only the latest news. For newcomers, readings can be assembled from material provided by the national Alzheimer's organization, Alzheimer's Disease and Related Disorders Association (ADRDA). These may be photocopies that the person can keep. A book list can be developed, or better yet, the group can chip in to purchase books to be loaned to group members. How-to manuals are available, offering help on various problems, as are case histories of individuals, and research reports, and other material. The leader can encourage members to watch for and clip any articles that can be copied and circulated. An information-lookout person could function as a sort of librarian. Outside speakers, such as physicians, researchers, nurses, and counselors, may be valuable local resources. At each meeting some educational material should be presented to keep members well informed. But repetition of the same information at meeting after meeting should be avoided. Instead, tell about research, an upcoming TV show, or a new book, etc. Basic information about community resources, legal advice on durable power of attorney, or day care centers, for example, could be compiled by a member or members, and given out to each newcomer. Adding to and updating local lists are a continuing need. Requests by members will provide ideas for programs in the area of information and assistance.

Another goal could be education for the community. A committee of members could plan news releases about the disease and its prevalence, the significance of support groups, and the need for understanding a patient's behavior in public. Public forums could be arranged. A high school assembly talk, or a meeting with a high school service club, or with nursing home staffs, all would help to widen understanding of the illness. This community education makes it easier for the caregiver and the patient to be respected and

understood by the residents of the town or the
neighborhood of the city in which they live.

Out of shared concerns and problems come the
feelings of empathy, understanding, and inspiration
for the members. At each meeting there must be the
time and the comfortable atmosphere that foster
openness in talking about whatever is on the
caregivers' minds. This unburdening and sharing is
the heart and soul of each support group. It must
be nourished and skillfully handled in order to
assure the continuation of the group as a meaning-
ful experience for each attendee. Caregivers feel
very isolated, sometimes even estranged from family
members. Their pride and self-respect often
constrains them from discussing unpleasantries with
friends. In the support group, they find sympathe-
tic responses, thus reducing their own stress and
anxiety. The reinforcement, encouragement, understanding, and sharing of survival techniques, all
develop bonds of friendship and affection for each
other.

Leaders can aid such bonding by various means.
Some suggestions include the following:

♦ Entry to the meetings should be pleasant:
soft background music, comfortable chairs, a non-
threatening atmosphere, a warm personal welcome as
a person enters the room; name tags; refreshments.
A show-and-tell object brought by a member, such as
a photograph or a letter from someone who has
helped. Minimize awkwardness.

♦ Seating should be casual, preferably in a
circle, if possible.

♦ Opening of the meeting by the leader should
be casual and warm, maybe humorous.

♦ Rounds (going around the circle asking questions) are particularly effective in getting groups
started and in helping the members learn about each
other and their circumstances. By using rounds,
the group leader can ask each member to identify
him- or herself, and state briefly the reason for
coming to the group and what he or she wants to get
out of it. Rounds are also used by the facilitator

to identify the specific circumstances and problems of the caregiver.

♦ The leader could begin rounds by telling a personal experience or that of a friend, then continuing to the next person. Leaders should also explain that this sharing is optional and those who don't feel like talking can "pass." At this point, it must be stated that these are to be brief reports, and that time is limited, so that each can have a turn within the time available (one hour perhaps). When an individual starts to dump years of problems, the leader can stem the flow of words by saying tactfully, "I'd like to talk with you later about that," or, "Let's get someone here who knows about that and they'll be able to help you-- after we get around the circle."

♦ The rounds can also include happy events for the caregiver, and pleasant surprises in the patient's behavior.

♦ Another technique is to separate people into diads, triads, or quads, with an old timer in each group. This gives more people more time to talk. The leader can go from group to group, and can be called over to a group which has a problem or needs another opinion.

♦ Sometimes groups may be subdivided by age, or by family relationships, and it may be helpful to have a small group of spouses meet separately from adult children who may be caregivers, since their feelings and concerns may be different as their role in the family is different.

♦ The facilitator can explain listening skills to help the members learn to concentrate on what the speaker is saying instead of the listener thinking of a response to what is being said. One way is to paraphrase the statement the person just made. A third person can be a coach/referee to see if the message gets across.

The above are some suggestions that have proved helpful. The list is not exhaustive. New ideas will develop to meet the needs of different groups.

II. Bringing out the Best

Self-disclosure can be very difficult for some people. A supportive group leader can be helpful in facilitating that activity. The leader might read excerpts from The Transparent Self, by Sidney Jourard, to emphasize the physical and mental values of discussing feelings and problems. The ability to disclose feelings and problems will usually develop after a person has attended a few meetings, but only if the atmosphere is warm and supportive.

Relationships with family members can become strained, adversarial, or even broken over the matter of the patient's illness, or the choice of caregiver, or the methods of caregiving. Loss of those ties is grievous to the patient and the caregiver. The arguing is irksome and even worse is an added burden on the caregiver. The leader can start a discussion of this problem. Probably the conclusion will be that the relative or friend misunderstands the nature of Alzheimer's disease. They have no realization that the patient can often rise to the occasion when friends are visiting, so that all appears well to the outsider who wonders what the caregiver's fuss is about. The leader can suggest ways to promote understanding, for example, by having a relative or relatives care for the patient over a weekend, or having them read a book, such as The 36-Hour Day, by Nancy Mace and Peter Rabins, or having them visit a support group meeting. Usually, when they understand the caregiver's problems fully, plus when they view the patient's worsening condition, this will help heal the rift. Otherwise, a counselor will be needed to intervene with the family.

Friends sometimes drop away, which is another loss for the caregiver. As that happens, the support group becomes more valuable since members understand each other's problems. Social occasions for the group, sometimes including the patients,

are helpful for friendships and for maintaining the
vitality of the group. By planning picnics, potluck
dinners, and other special social occasions, the
group reinforces its structure as a unit that is
both helpful and pleasurable.

The psychological needs of the group members
usually relate to understanding and handling of the
patient's behavior.   As the mind deteriorates,
hallucinations, paranoia, difficulty in communicating, perseveration, and loss of motor skills,
all tax the caregiver's ability to understand and
to cope.   The group leader can suggest that a
person with a good sound mind should be skillful
enough to cope with the failing mind's bizarre
responses, behaviors, and statements.

The leader can suggest that the caregiver
assess the patient's positive attributes--what
things can the patient still do or understand; then
suggest that the caregiver let the patient do those
things, rather than teaching him or her greater
helplessness. A real situation can be set up to
role-play, and the group can discuss the logic best
suited to handle it. A program of vignettes (of a
variety of problem situations) can be used as a
basis for a psychological analysis.   Tapes are
usually available from the local ADRDA office.

A counselor can be helpful in explaining the
difficulties   of   dealing   with   a   neurological
handicap. With Alzheimer's patients, for example,
it is usually futile to try to get them to see
reality as the rational caregiver does.   Often it
is preferable to agree, to go along with the
erroneous or even the fantasies, then to distract
and divert them into another activity.   Reality
therapy does not work.   Other psychological needs
and problems could be discussed by a mental health
panel at a group meeting.

The leader can suggest also that caregivers
speak of "my patient" rather than "my husband" or
"my mother," especially when the change in personality of the patient is so great that he or she has
become "someone I once knew" to the caregiver.

Developing and keeping some detachment from the patient is helpful to the caregiver in dealing with emotions.

The caregiver's emotional rollercoaster of ups and downs, anger and remorse, frustration and satisfaction, needs to be handled by the leader in a clinical mode, as prevention before the need. The emotions of caregiving can be explained and then discussed by the group. For instance, what is happening to the caregiver who responds to the patient impulsively, angrily, inappropriately? Has the caregiver forgotten that the patient is mentally out of control? Each caregiver could write down afterward what the emotional storm was all about. This can be done at the support group meeting. The leader can then make a suggestion that each member try keeping a journal until the next meeting. The journal can deal primarily with feelings, the events that trigger them, and the responses, verbal and physical. A counselor at the next meeting could lead a discussion of what triggers the strong emotions. Caregivers may discover that keeping a journal is helpful in venting emotions and in diffusing them the next time.

Dealing with the emotions of grieving can sometimes be best helped by a closed group of six or so caregivers who find their feelings of sadness are adding greatly to their caregiving burden. Suggestions from a professional counselor would include the steps in the grieving process to be discussed. Group members might also write a life history of the patient. Reliving pleasant memories can create a happiness that so many good things have happened in the patient's life. By doing this in a closed group, where a time commitment of at least four sessions is made, the caregivers may avoid a harmful depression. Emotions are strongly felt by caregivers and they must be skillfully dealt with or they will cause serious debilities, such as ulcers and other disabling illnesses.

Caregivers must also look ahead to the time when the burden becomes too great and more daily help is necessary. The group leader is wise to make contact with nearby community resources. A nursing home administrator or group home leader might be invited to address the support group. A visit to a care facility might be arranged. Most families are very reluctant to transfer the care-giving function to an institution. With greater knowledge of their problems and procedures, many will develop a degree of admiration for the professionals. This decision-making process can be greatly facilitated when the caregiver shares it with the group.

Caregiving does not cease when the patient is placed in a nursing home. At first the relief from burden is a real release from bondage. Many nursing homes suggest that the caregiver not visit during the first two weeks. This gives separation a good start, respite for the caregiver, and acclimatization for the patient. But after the first feelings of freedom, the caregiver may experience a tremendous sense of loss, followed by remorse and guilt over unfinished business with the patient. Those feelings of, "I could have done better," "I shouldn't have been so impatient," etc., can be depressing and debilitating. The support group is needed at this time to affirm the caregivers' worth and pride, and to reassure them that these feelings will lessen. The caregiver is encouraged to remain in the support group to help others. This is also good therapy for the care-giver. Reports at rounds will enable him or her to share experiences from visits to the institution and the status of the patient.

At the time of the patient's death, the support group's strength is needed to help with autopsy arrangements, if the patient's brain is donated to research. The procedures would have been explained in the group meeting programs, but the bereaved caregiver still needs help. Knowing about something in advance is one thing, dealing with it when it happens is another.

After the death of the patient, or when any member feels a grievous sense of loss, a closed small group of people could meet for four or six sessions with someone to lead them through the process of grief. The leader should be a trained person so that the group will go beyond the tears and tissue stage. Rebuilding one's life can be helped by helping others. The bereaved caregiver's experience can be used to help others, with the person acting either as a group leader or as a consultant.

Group cohesion and a sense of unity can also be fostered by making the group meeting both a time for problem solving and a time for relaxation and enjoyment. Refreshments can be served at the end of the meeting to give an opportunity for the members to enjoy each other's company. Humor is not only fun, but also a therapeutic addition to the meetings or the social gatherings. Some groups have developed a joke-swapping format to structure humor into the meetings. The process of taking care of someone with Alzheimer's disease can be so overwhelming that the caregiver forgets that there can still be laughter and humor in the world, even though they are removed from it on a daily basis.

There will be times when the group will want to have a lecture on a given topic, such as the financial and legal implications of Alzheimer's disease. Or, there may be times when the group may meet with a larger group on an issue of care and treatment, or on nutrition concerns. Case studies are sometimes useful tools for understanding the disease as well. A case study not only provides information, but also illuminates certain aspects of care and arrangements that may not yet have surfaced in the regular meetings. These variations of format will help keep the group stimulating.

The group leader should also anticipate the need for meeting with some members of the group individually to assist them through a crisis or particularly burdensome time. Group members will go through various peaks and valleys during the

process of care, sometimes their needs are so
overwhelming that they cannot be adequately
addressed in the group. The group leader should be
able to identify community resources that can
assist the person through a difficult period. The
leader and certain members of the group may also be
called upon to meet separately with one of the
members, as well to serve as peer counselors.

The group may grow to a size that is unwieldy
and impossible for a participatory format. Then is
the time to split, with a core of old timers to
share the start of the splinter group. The size is
not determined by membership lists alone, but by
attendance lists that are taken at each meeting.
An attendance average of more than twenty people
should start the leader planning a future split.

The place of meeting may need to be changed.
Most groups have found it best not to meet in
members' homes since that may produce added stress
to the caregiver. When attendance lags, a
telephone network can be useful in identifying the
reasons for absence. Problems may be worked out at
the group meeting or over the phone. Newspaper
announcements may bring in new members.

However, the best way to maintain the group,
to give it lasting life, is to set goals (revising
when appropriate) and target those goals, giving
priority to the majority needs of the members. The
format for the meeting can have something for
almost everyone: a warm welcome, rounds for getting
acquainted with caregivers and their burdens,
informational update on research and news, a brief
presentation and discussion on one of the common
concerns, a show-and-tell time on the good and
happy happenings, some problem-solving (this must
not be too time-consuming, either a pre-set time
limit, or assign helpers "who can help Barbara with
her car-driving problem," "Ralph needs to know how
to get a durable power of attorney--can anybody
help?"), and affirmations and good-bye until the
next time.

The group leader can also use the group process and the group history to assess periodically what the individual members and the group as a whole have learned about the caregiving process. The group and the individual now have a history and valuable experience; they have learned how to reflect on their situation, analyze it, and examine their lives and needs in different ways than they would have imagined possible at the beginning. They have synthesized information, generalized about it, and applied it to their daily lives; they have had an opportunity to evaluate the effectiveness of the solutions that were identified.

And, they have survived and are surviving the caregiving process, and have learned that the strengths they have gained can be applied to all areas of their lives, and that they can cope and survive with strength and dignity.

Suggested Readings

Davis, Bruce.   The Magical Child within You. Millbrae, CA.: Celestial Arts, 1977.

Heston, Leonard, and June A. White. Dementia. New York: W.H. Freeman & Co., 1983.

Ivey, Allen E., and Norma B. Gluckstern.   Basic Attending Skills.   North Amherst, MA.: Microtraining Associates, Inc., 1978.

Jourard, Sidney M.   The Transparent Self.   New York: Van Nostrand Co., 1971.

Mace, Nancy, and Peter Rabin.   The 36-Hour Day. Baltimore, MD.: Johns Hopkins University Press, 1981.

Otten, Jane, and Florence Shelley.   When Your Parents Grow Old.   New York: New American Library, 1978.

Reisberg, Barry.   A Guide to Alzheimer's Disease. New York: Free Press, 1983.

Satir, Virginia.   Self Esteem.   Millbrae, CA.: Celestial Arts, 1975.

Families and the Fragmented Service Delivery System

Pamela A. Sisson and Paula Gilbreath

This chapter addresses some of the technical issues faced by families caring for Alzheimer's patients. In addition to the practical difficulties associated with any illness, the nature of this disease contributes to family stress. That stress is often aggravated by the fragmented social and health service delivery system, as well as by the legal and financial questions that the family must settle.

In the beginning of the disease process, family members typically deny the new and strange behaviors of a family member. The family is often confused and uncertain about what to do, and its members are usually hesitant to admit that there is a problem. When the problem can no longer be ignored, the step is finally taken to see a physician, who may give a preliminary diagnosis of Alzheimer's disease. Frequently the family is told to wait and see what happens and to return in six months or so if the behavior is getting worse. The family is in a state of limbo while waiting for the disease to progress.

The family may seek a second opinion to make certain that Alzheimer's disease is the correct diagnosis. This is, in fact, one of the things they should do. It is essential that the family consult with a knowledgeable physician or team of professionals to prevent misdiagnosis, and make certain a complete and thorough physical and psychological exam is given to the patient. Part 1 of this volume outlines the various tests that should be administered to ascertain most accurately if a person has Alzheimer's disease.

As the disease progresses, the caregiver may become more and more isolated. Frequently, friends and non-caregiving family members will avoid both the patient and caregiver because the patient's "strange" behavior is difficult for many people to tolerate. The caregiver is often totally immersed in day-to-day care and continually confined to the home.

Caregivers need to identify the available resources in their community at the earliest possible time, and then plan ways in which these existing services can assist them in their care-giving task. But caregivers often do not know where to turn to find services and, in many cases, do not know that there are any services available. This chapter will suggest ways to find community services, and delineate some the financial and legal issues that families must confront during the course of this most difficult of diseases.

Community Resources

How do families find services? Often their first contact is with a physician, who may or may not know much about the existing service delivery system. Depending on the size of the community, there may or may not be a local chapter of the Alzheimer's Disease and Related Disorders Association (ADRDA) or an independent support group which the family can approach for information and help. Until faced with caring for a chronically impaired member, many families do not know that there are organizations like ADRDA, that there are adult day centers, or that there are "chore" and other in-home services available to them. Simply stated, most families gain access to services through desperate necessity and in a random fashion. Only by finding one critical agency or organization, do they learn about the existence of many supportive community services. When they do finally gain access to services, they also learn that the system designed to give assistance is fragmented, complex, and fraught with duplications and gaps.

How can families be helped through the mire of the current delivery system? One of the easiest first steps is for an organization or agency to compile information about the services it offers, and the eligibility requirements for those services. For those agencies and organizations to be of real use to the family, the individuals within each organization must also be knowledgeable about other formal services in addition to their own. They must be able to see how their service fits into the larger service delivery system. Agency personnel should not only know about the aging-network (e.g., area agencies on aging), but also be familiar with the services available through the Veterans Administration, mental health, medical, and legal service systems, including eligibility information.

Ideally, each organization should be able to provide the names of other agencies and organizations that offer services for which families may be eligible. For example, an Area Agency on Aging (AAA) might not list just all of its own contracted services, but also those of other agencies, such as those available through the Veterans Administration and the mental health networks. Since more than direct service needs are involved for families who are caring for someone with Alzheimer's disease, lists of legal services, support groups, hospices, and nursing homes can be of immense value. If agency personnel are not aware of or familiar with these other services, then they will experience great difficulty in assisting a family to meet its needs.

A knowledge of services outside the formal service delivery system can be important as well. Many support groups, adult day care, and respite programs are offered by church groups, community colleges, or local schools, as well as by such service organizations as the Kiwanis or Elks. Thus, families should also contact service agencies, churches, and libraries if information about informal community resources was not obtained through their contacts with direct service groups. In more rural and remote areas where people live at greater distances from each other, government agencies such as the Post Office can be instrumental in connecting people to programs that provide assistance, or in informing service agencies about apparent changes in the home environment. Hospitals can also be useful in providing information about community services.

There are many options for exploring and developing community resources. In each community it is essential that the agencies working with families and caregivers of Alzheimer's patients be willing to serve as brokers for referring families to appropriate help, and to work with other groups and agencies to develop assistance responsive to the needs of the families in that community. Obviously, a program that is effective in New York City may not be one that would meet the needs of a small, isolated rural community. The availability and structure of services and programs should reflect the particular character of the community being served. Sometimes individual initiative is required to develop needed support group services.

Legal and Financial Issues

Some of the immediate problems facing the family of an Alzheimer's patient involve legal and financial affairs. Because the disease leads to a progressive decline of mental functioning, there comes a point in the disease when the Alzheimer victim is no longer considered to be legally competent. Unfortunately, this is an issue many families either overlook or do not consider until it is too late to seek relatively simple legal remedies. As soon as possible after diagnosis, steps need to be taken to insure that the legal and financial affairs of the afflicted person will be managed by someone who is legally competent. Some of the more simple steps may include closing joint checking accounts, transferring funds, and preparing or updating a will. There can often be problems with creditors, since patients may forget that they even have bills to pay. Some individuals afflicted with Alzheimer's disease start giving things away to strangers, not knowing what they are doing.

At some stage of the disease, the issue of guardianship or conservatorship usually arises: who will be legally responsible to act for the patient when he or she can no longer make decisions about care or daily activities? The sooner a family faces this issue the better. Lack of attention can lead to disastrous consequences.

Legal issues. Legal advice should be sought as soon as possible. State laws vary so extensively that it is possible here only to outline some of the more general problems and their solutions. Agencies may be able to help the family identify lawyers who are knowledgeable about issues such as guardianship, conservatorship, and durable power of attorney. The precise management of legal affairs will vary from family to family. The arrangements that are made when a spouse is caring for the Alzheimer patient will differ significantly from arrangements made when an adult child or other family member is caring for the patient. Legal issues such as these are difficult to face at the beginning of the disease, but the consequences of not doing so can be significant. If the patient is still legally competent to participate, this will assist the process of deciding the legal and fiscal responsibilities for caregiver. In some cases families as a whole decide. If no prior provisions are made, often a court assigns the caregiving role and the legal and fiscal responsibilities.

What are some of these legal options available to families? They include power of attorney, durable power of attorney, conservatorship, living trusts and guardianships. It is important that these possibilities be discussed early in the disease process and with the patient, if possible, so that he or she can participate in deciding on the care plan and the disposition of possessions and funds. If Alzheimer's victims are mentally capable, they should be involved in making decisions that will affect them the rest of their lives, even though at some point they will no longer remember they have made such arrangements.

Durable power of attorney. Durable power of attorney can be an essential designation for families caring for Alzheimer's patients. It is often suggested that one or two people should hold it. Durable power of attorney, unlike power of attorney, does not need to be renewed and does not require that the person (the patient) delegating authority remain mentally competent. Power of attorney, on the other hand, usually requires periodic renewal and that the person making that designation be mentally competent at the time of renewal. Thus, durable power of attorney often fits the realistic circumstances of families caring for someone with Alzheimer's disease. In brief, durable power of attorney remains in effect during the patient's incompetency, while power of attorney is voided when a patient becomes mentally incompetent.

The person holding a durable power of attorney is in a powerful position in that he or she is, in fact, acting as the person represented. The holder may make financial and medical decisions, decisions about physical care or living arrangements of the patient. Durable power of attorney can be restricted to issues of health care, so that when the patient can no longer give informed consent, the person designated can do so. Because the durable power of attorney is such a powerful role, the person or persons playing that role must be trusted completely by the family and the patient.

Families should discuss with knowledgeable lawyers the intricacies of durable power of attorney. Depending upon how the document is drafted, there may be taxation issues associated with it, since the managed funds may be counted as income in some cases. A durable power of attorney may begin immediately after execution, or may be

postponed until such time as several other people
state in writing that the individual has lost his
or her mental competency.   Courts do have the
power, if petitioned, to appoint a conservator or
guardian who can override the durable power of
attorney.

Laws vary extensively from state to state, and
laws change frequently.   Families need to consult
an attorney as soon as possible to learn what
options are available in their particular state and
for their specific situation.   No one solution will
fit all people.

Conservatorship or guardianship.   A conservatorship or, in some states, a guardianship can be
established for patients with Alzheimer's disease.
Arrangements can vary from managing the person's
estate to personal care of the patient.   In order
to have someone placed involuntarily in an institution, such as a nursing home, a conservator or
guardian must be named.   This is a court appointed
position for which the patient or family members or
friends must make legal petition.   It must be
demonstrated at a hearing that the person is no
longer capable of self-care.

Sometimes conservatorships are limited to
management of the patient's assets.   The conservator manages the patient's property, pays the bills,
and manages the income or trust account that may
have been created.   In many cases, the conservator
is accountable to the court for expenditures and
management of the patient's assets.

Financial Considerations

Intimately related to the legal issues are the
financial issues.   Alzheimer's disease is not an
"official" disease.   It is part of a broader
diagnosis of senile dementia.   Frequently the
consequences of this are that Alzheimer's disease
is covered by Medicare only if a patient is
admitted to a skilled nursing facility.   Even then,

Medicare coverage is usually limited to twenty-seven days.

Families are eligible for Medicaid support only if they "pauperize" themselves, that is, "spend down" or exhaust their financial resources and become financially eligible for Medicaid.

Since long-term custodial nursing home care is not covered by Medicare, and nursing homes cost about $1,500 to $2,000 monthly, most families simply cannot afford such care. Additionally, some states do not have community property laws so families must act to divide family assets or risk spending all assets for the care of one spouse with the result that the surviving spouse is rendered penniless. In some extraordinarily painful cases, happily married spouses have been forced to seek divorce to protect the family house and other assets by dividing the property.

If there are sufficient family resources, it may be advisable for the family to discuss setting up a living trust. This type of trust can be used to protect property, avoid taxes and probate, and ensure that there are funds available that can be used for the patient's care. It can also be used to prevent the patient from mismanaging his or her financial affairs. The living trust is normally managed by the conservator or the guardian.

These issues should also be raised at the earliest possible time with a lawyer familiar with tax laws and estate planning. Trusts and other financial arrangements have the financial well-being of the individual and the family at stake, so they should be done carefully and precisely. If patients are still in the early stages of the disease, they can participate in the decision-making process so that they know they will be cared for by someone who loves them and cares about their emotional and physical well-being.

There are few uniform laws from state to state about financial issues and property. There are no two family circumstances that are absolutely identical. It is essential that families contact an attorney well versed in these issues as soon as possible so that they have an opportunity to consider the various alternatives that are available to them and to be able to anticipate some of the legal and financial consequences of the disease.

Agency personnel can play a key role in assisting families in understanding the laws in their state, and in guiding them to reputable lawyers, law firms, or legal services agencies.

In-home Versus Institutional Care Options

The majority of Alzheimer's patients are cared for in their own home or in the home of a family member. Home care is difficult and often over-whelming to the caregiver. An Alzheimer's victim can be transformed from a person known and loved to a shell of the former self. The person may look the same, but everything else has changed. A patient may engage in endless, non-stop chattering; another might wander or become violent; still others may engage in totally inappropriate social and/or sexual behavior.

Coupled with the progressive change and loss of personality is the unrelenting physical decline. A patient will reach a stage when he or she can no longer get dressed, eat, or remember to perform personal hygiene. Eventually many patients must be watched constantly so they do not wander from home or do things to endanger themselves or others.

There often comes a point when the in-home caregiver usually must consider some alternate living arrangements. This may mean hiring someone to provide in-home care, finding an adult foster home or other facilities that can accommodate Alzheimer's patients, or choosing nursing home care. In some communities there may be several choices depending on a family's income and the size of the community. In some areas there will be few choices, and the choices to be made may seem extreme. In addition to organized housing, such as

nursing homes, some churches have facilities that
may be available. It is essential that agencies
work with families to determine their needs,
assets, and emotional and physical resources in
order to assist them in identifying ways to meet
the on-going care needs of the patient.

Family Participation in Caregiving and Decision-making

The ways in which families make decisions about the
care of an Alzheimer's patient will vary as the
structure and relationships within each family
vary. It is a difficult time for every family
member, and the decisions that have to be made can
exacerbate family jealousies; questions about
finances and family inheritances can arise, perhaps
especially in the case of stepparents and step-
children. Some families flock together; others do
not.
    While it is important that agency personnel
not get into the middle of these frays, it would be
useful for the family if the agency could put them
in touch with such groups as ADRDA, since support
groups can assist individuals in facing some of the
problems and in finding resources to address those
problems. Support group advice might include
suggestions to see counselors and/or lawyers or
other professionals.
    In summary, the best way that organizations
and agencies can assist families is to understand
the problems that families face--legal, financial,
emotional, and physical--and be able to refer them
to services that give them some sense of control
over their situation. Service providers will be
most effective if they know the myriad services
that are available and can anticipate the types of
problems that families will encounter. Alzheimer's
disease is not the same as a stroke. It is
progressive, and as it progresses, it will drain
families emotionally, financially, and physically
unless they know where to turn for aid and support.

Reference

Roach, Marianne. Another Name for Madness.   Boston: Houghton Mifflin, 1985.

Starting a Support Group
Case Histories

Kathleen O'Connor
with Deborah Anderson, Judy Gellatly, Jane Schmidt, and Doris Weaver

Support groups are a major help to caregivers of Alzheimer's patients. Most caregivers are home-bound and often suffer intense feelings of isolation. They frequently believe they are the only ones faced with such heavy daily responsibilities. As the disease progresses, caregivers can become increasingly isolated as friends and family stop visiting. Joining or forming support groups can help enormously in overcoming feelings of isolation and hopelessness.

The support groups for Alzheimer's disease that are best known are those associated with the Alzheimer's Disease and Related Disorders Association (ADRDA). This organization not only disseminates information about the disease but also stimulates public awareness of the nature of the disease and its problems. It also supports research efforts to investigate the cause, cure, and effective treatment for this dehumanizing illness. One of the hallmark activities of ADRDA, however, is its support of the caregiver, which is most widely seen in the form of support groups. These groups not only provide moral support and reassurance, but also are a forum for exchanging information. They have been almost universally acknowledged as one of the most effective forms of assistance for caregivers.

Although ADRDA and similar organizations sponsor support groups, there are many communities where support groups do not exist. One of the goals of this section is to describe the various ways in which support groups can be formed and the many purposes they can serve. Some support groups

have been started by a few concerned individuals in
the community, others have developed by focusing
the efforts of existing groups, while still others
were initiated by an institution or by agency staff
members who recognized a need for some sort of
support for Alzheimer's caregivers.   There is no
one "right" way to start a support group.   The kind
of group that develops depends on community
resources, the skills and interests of the group
members, the size of the community, and the availability of professionals who could be called upon
to provide assistance.

This section outlines the experiences of
several different support groups in terms of how
they were started, how they were organized, and how
they carried out their functions.   The structure
and functions of the groups varied as their development varied.   The tone of the initial group was
often set by the personal style and interests of
the group leader or organizer.   The common element
in all these experiences, however, was the effort
to develop a program that met the needs of the
caregivers.   Meeting these different needs often
meant that the original structure and purpose of
the group evolved over time as new members came
into the group, as one of the original leaders
left, and as the needs of the members changed
during the course of the disease.

The examples presented here demonstrate how
support groups can be formed by individuals or by
institutional representatives.   They also show how
groups will function differently given local
resources and availability of professional support.
One support group was located in a primarily
agricultural community with little professional
support, while another was initiated in an urban
area with a major academic health center and
extensive community resources.   Others were started
in rural and suburban centers with active agency
participation.

Grass Roots Organizing
with Betty Jane Schmidt

The first group history is based on the experiences
of Betty Jane Schmidt who lives in Wenatchee,
Washington, a city of 35,000 people. Wenatchee is
located equidistant between the two major population centers of Washington State, Seattle and
Spokane. It has an Area Agency on Aging, a mental
health clinic, a hospital, community college, and
library, one hundred and fifty service organizations, and fifty churches and synagogues.

Organizer's background. When Schmidt started
the support group, her husband had been a patient
since 1980 in a nursing home facility at Veterans
Administration (VA) Medical Center nearly three
hundred miles away in the Seattle-Tacoma Metropolitan Area. Prior to his admission at the VA, she
cared for him at home for a year and a half after
he had been forced to take an early retirement. In
1972 he was diagnosed as having the disease.

When Schmidt realized that she no longer could
care for her husband at home, she felt depressed
and alone. She soon discovered, however, that she
knew two other women in her community, Elsie Havers
and Nancy Wiley, who were in similar circumstances.
When they found each other, they "weren't all alone
out in the wilderness." They joined together and
decided that there were probably more people than
they realized in the community who were in similar
situations. Feeling the need to help, they decided
to form a support group.

Initial Meetings

Through the generosity of a friend of Havers'
Schmidt obtained a brief videotaped presentation
about family caregiving. She put a notice in the
local newspaper about a "non-sponsored" meeting on
Alzheimer's disease. The three organizers were
uncertain how many people, if any, would come. "We
originally thought that if we got twelve people, we

would be doing well," Schmidt said. "Fifty people showed up. We were overwhelmed."

The first thing they did at the meeting was to get everyone's name, address, and telephone number by passing around a sheet of paper on a clipboard. The three organizers then discussed the relief they had felt in finding each other, the problems they faced, and the isolation they had formerly felt in caring for spouses and family members. At the end of the meeting, the people present urged Schmidt and her friends to organize another meeting soon so they could continue to meet. Instead of choosing a place that might produce anxiety in some members, such as a hospital or a nursing home or church, they decided to have the second meeting in the library of one of the city's elementary schools.

During the second meeting, they distributed blank sheets of paper and asked the participants to list the problems of caregiving that they faced every day. Schmidt took these lists home and organized the problems into categories. "I was absolutely amazed at how every list was practically the same. We held another meeting to discuss the problems and that's how we got started."

Schmidt, Wiley, and Havers did not want to start a group simply for the sake of starting a group. But according to Schmidt, "one of the things I realized after my husband was in a nursing home, is that I had practically killed myself in the process of caring for him at home. It took me three years from the time he was institutionalized to regain my energy. I was concerned that other people were doing the same thing. Something had to be done."

This initial support group worked closely with existing local resources. A file on Alzheimer's disease was established at the local library. The file included information about the disease, lists of reference books, and the names and telephone numbers of people caregivers could call for various types of assistance. "This is extremely valuable," Schmidt says. "I get calls at home from people in very stressful situations. These people often don't know where to turn."

Organizing suggestions. An important feature of support groups is that they are not static. They evolve as the needs of the individuals in the group evolve. Schmidt emphasizes the importance of having a strong core for a group to survive. These key individuals come and go. Depending on the level of stress at home, they may attend all the meetings in order to help themselves get by, but as things calm down, they may not attend. Having a solid core is essential, therefore, if there is going to be continuity to the group.

Larger communities have more ready access to professionals who can help form that core. The Wenatchee group did not have such a resource available at the time that it was forming. Schmidt thinks it would have been useful to have someone serve as a resource person who could have helped the group organize. The group still exists, how-ever, and is still functioning effectively. It is composed largely of individuals who are fulltime caregivers or people who are working fulltime to pay for care for their spouse or parent. These fulltime commitments do not leave much time for community organizing, Schmidt feels, nor time for the much needed public relations and information sharing that is helpful to those just learning about the disease. Having professionals associated with other agencies could be very helpful in getting notices on television or radio or even placing articles in the local newspaper.

Time is a major factor, especially for volun-teers who are fulltime caregivers or fulltime employees, not to mention bearing the stress of responsibilities. Schmidt's time was not her own even when she was no longer in a daily caregiving role. She had to return to work full time since all the funds she and her husband had accumulated toward retirement had been exhausted in paying for his care prior to his admission to a Veterans Administration facility.

A recurring theme in support groups is that members must be able to express their feelings. "Probably the single most important function of the leaders," according to Schmidt, "is to expose their feelings and thereby give permission to others to do so. If they can show the anger and frustration they have felt, and acknowledge that their behavior is not always what they would want it to be, and that sometimes daily stresses just creep up and they lose control, then others will feel more comfortable to do the same."

The sensitivity of the group leader and members is another important factor in keeping a support group going. Schmidt calls it the ability to be a "shock absorber": "Caregivers face very real frustrations and often delicate, intimate problems. What do you do with a spouse who is sexually stimulated, but who can't talk or is incontinent? How do you handle a loved one who is violent? I have seen people with broken fingers and broken ribs. These forums have to be a place to help."

Another continuing source of tension that support groups can assist with is the relationship between the caregiver and the other family members. The group and the group leader can offer help when family members have conflicting views about the disease. Meetings outside the support group can frequently help families recognize that their situation is not unique and that they are not having unusual reactions. Schmidt has found that having the group leader meet with a family can often permit the family members to vent feelings. These meetings also help those who are denying that there is a problem learn about the difficulty of the caregiving situation and recognize the tremendous stress faced by the caregiver.

Finally, Schmidt finds leadership to be a key issue in keeping a support group going. The support group is a very intense emotional and physical experience. "Burn-out" among leaders can be a real problem. Having a rotating leadership helps, Schmidt has found, as well as having other members of the committee serve in different roles, such as a program chairman or a public relations person.

The experience of Schmidt, Havers, and Wiley serves as a useful guide on how to develop and stimulate the creation of a group with individual commitment and energy and few community resources. The experience of another, more urban group illustrates a quite different approach not only because of the differences in the origin of the group but also because of the differences in the availability of community resources.

Converging Interest Groups
with Judy Gellatly

Judy Gellatly is a co-founder and leader of a support group for Alzheimer's caregivers in the suburbs east of Seattle. The entire metropolitan area has a population exceeding one million, and has a vast array of medical services, hospitals, clinics, and community services available to Alzheimer patients and families. One example is the University of Washington and its Health Sciences Center where the faculty are actively involved in research on the diagnosis, assessment, care, and treatment of Alzheimer's disease.

Organizer's background. Gellatly's husband was diagnosed as having Alzheimer's disease in 1972. After his diagnosis they went to a special clinic associated with the University Hospital, the Geriatric and Family Services Clinic, and made the commitment to do whatever they could to combat Alzheimer's disease.

Initial Phase

In 1977, there were no support groups in the Seattle area for the hundreds of caregivers managing patients with Alzheimer's disease. But, while those caregivers felt alone and isolated, there were many converging activities that resulted in the formation of support groups in the Seattle Metropolitan Area.

In 1978, the University of Washington opened its Geriatric and Family Services Clinic, founded and directed by Dr. Burton Reifler, Associate Professor, Department of Psychiatry and Behavioral Sciences. Comprehensive diagnostic procedures were developed and caregivers were educated on the many facets of supportive management for their patients. Research on the impact of the illness on family members was also being conducted in the Veteran's Administration Medical Center in Seattle. Dr. Monte Scott, a resident in psychiatry, assembled a group of caregivers who were referred by local physicians and who had spouses and/or parents with Alzheimer's disease.

Gellatly, whose husband had been diagnosed at the Geriatric and Family Services Clinic, was part of that initial group. She says of the early meetings, "We were all strangers to each other. We were given a box of Kleenex and told to talk about our patients' behaviors and our feelings and our problems. We became acquainted with each other, first with name tags, later through each other's burdens. We talked about superficial problems, mundane things at first. Then, with trust and confidentiality, we found we could disclose and talk about anything. We used lots of tissue."

By the time Dr. Scott's research project ended, twelve sessions later, the caregivers did not want to disband. They said, "We've learned so much from each other. We've risked disclosing our innermost feelings. We've spoken of the unspeakable in our patient's behavior." In other words, the group had become, with only minimal guidance from Dr. Scott who kept them on track, a full-fledged mutual support group. The group voted unanimously to continue meeting independently.

Simultaneously, another group had been formed through the Geriatric Research Education and Clinical Center (GRECC) at the Veterans Administration Medical Center in American Lake. This group was composed of wives whose veteran husbands were patients of the VA. This group also met over the course of the year and had come to rely on those meetings for information and support. The group in Tacoma called itself A.S.I.S.T. for Alzheimer's Support, Information and Service Team.

The two groups began to meet together and finally merged and incorporated as a non-profit educational foundation. It became the nucleus of a state-wide network of forty plus support groups. The original Seattle area group elected a board that took the initiative in organizational issues. It established committees to help the support groups to function and grow geographically.

These groups in Seattle and Tacoma sent representatives to New York in 1978 to meet with eight others grassroots organizations. The meeting was convened to found and develop a national organization: Alzheimer's Disease and Related Disorders Association.

On-Going Efforts

Today, Gellatly, who is now a social worker and still a caregiver, continues to lead her support group near Seattle. These bi-monthly meetings follow the same format as that of the original 1978 research support group. The variations in the format and structure of the meeting come as a result of suggestions by the individual members. More materials are now available and presentations with videos, slides, and other special purpose meetings are held.

"Our group is open-ended so that the members attend when they can, when they feel the need for supportive others. Attendance varies more than in a closed group with a commitment to a definite number of members," according to Gellatly. Between meetings, counseling by the leader is available by telephone or home visits. Members have a telephone network to share and to encourage each other.

Gellatly's group has evolved since its inception. The changes reflect changes in the membership of the group and the evolving needs for support and problem solving. Knowledge of the illness has expanded, legislative issues have been addressed, and publicity about Alzheimer's has increased. The need for support groups, however, remains. Since the founding of that original group in 1978, over two hundred caregivers, patients and their families have been served, all by volunteer efforts. Gellatly's group is interesting in that it moved from information-sharing and problem-solving to incorporating into a non-profit organization that actively sponsored the growth of new support groups and dissemination of information to caregivers and the public about Alzheimer's disease. The model that this group developed is essentially the same structure used by other Alzheimer support groups. It was one of the pioneering efforts for Alzheimer's support groups in the country.

The group also demonstrates how support groups can evolve from other groups that initially had somewhat different intent or focus. While the initial impetus was a research project, the individuals in the group found meeting together extremely valuable in encouraging each other in their caregiving effort.

While the Seattle chapter had many resources available to it, and was assisted in the beginning by the medical community interested in a research project, the key ingredients remain individual commitment and concern.

Agency Sponsored or Initiated Groups
with Deborah Anderson and Doris Weaver

The two previous case histories focused on groups that were started by caregivers. Schmidt and her associates started by putting an ad in the paper. While the group started by Gellatly and others had been at one time formally associated with a research project at the University of Washington, the impetus to keep the group going came from Gellatly and other concerned caregivers. There are instances, however, where professionals affiliated with institutions see the need for a support group in a given community and play an instrumental role in gathering together a group of people with common concerns.

Doris Weaver is Director of Aging Services for Good Samaritan Hospital and Mental Health Center in Puyallup, Washington. Puyallup is a rural community of 173,000 citizens. The Good Samaritan Hospital provides a continuum of long-term care services with the community as well as serves as a service subcontractor with the local Area Agency on Aging in the county. In her work with individuals and families in the community, Weaver saw individual caregivers facing similar problems and perceived the need for a caregivers' support group in the immediate area. She remains actively involved in both building and maintaining support groups.

Weaver stresses that one of the differences between support groups developed by individuals in the community and agency personnel is the issue of who defines the focus. It is also important to determine the motive of the institution when an organization is instrumental in initiating a support group, or has a facilitator initiate and work with a support group. "There may be cases, for example," Weaver points out, "where nursing home staff may think that it would be 'useful' to have a support group for family members of Alzheimer's patients. But, the definition of usefulness must be defined. Is the group to serve the agency because someone in the agency thought it would be 'nice' to have a group as part of its program, or will the group assist in helping the staff work more effectively with the families?"

Like Schmidt and Gellatly, Weaver stresses that the support group must meet the needs of the caregivers. The members must believe that their own needs are being satisfied and that the group is not just meeting an undefined agency need for community interaction.

The two kinds of professionals that are most often involved in identifying the need for support groups, Weaver reports, are physicians and service providers. These individuals often perceive the need for a group because they see so many people who share similar problems. Again, the consumers of the group, the members, must see a need for it as well. Unless they do, the group will not be a success, no matter how well intentioned the creators were. The group must still focus on the practical needs of its members. "Unless it does so," says Weaver, "attendance will be sporadic and the group will not develop the stability and continuity necessary for its success."

There is often a delicate balance when an agency starts and/or provides continuing support for a group. It is not uncommon at the beginning for the group members to be uncertain about what they really need or want. The members are often frustrated, unhappy, and overwhelmed by their particular caregiving experience. Weaver stresses that a professional facilitator can be instrumental in easing this difficult phase for the group by helping the members focus on immediate problems that they can solve. "The facilitator must be able to make contacts, start a group, develop an informal agenda and provide the kernal to let the group develop. After that, the group must be able to define itself. Successful groups develop in similar ways: that is to say, they meet the needs of the members."

Weaver has also seen groups that started by themselves seek to attract professional assistance once the group is established. The reason most freqently given is that having a professional from an agency available to the group gives it some back-up during a period of transition in leadership within the group. Additionally, the professional can be instrumental in identifying experts from the community who may know something about particular problems, such as nutrition or legal issues. Often the professional can serve as a link to administrative help, such as assisting in reserving meeting rooms and helping with publicity for a major event sponsored by the group.

An important role for support groups that Weaver sees is the question of advocacy. The individuals facing the daily problems of caregiving have a more immediate understanding of the kinds of services that are necessary to support their effort as caregivers. The advocacy role of the individual members can be an important one in terms of gaining access to services. "Agencies cannot always serve as advocates since they are only one part of a larger budget request and service system," Weaver points out. "While the services that the agency requests may be important in meeting the needs of the community, legislators usually regard requests for additional funds or services as self-serving."

In addition, the professional leader or the facilitator can be of assistance in linking individuals and agencies with common concerns. Weaver suggests that if a nursing home is proposing to put up a new building in a community, the facilitator can work to bridge the gap between the people who are building the facility and the families who may place their members there. "The facilitator can arrange for the architect, for example, to attend a support group meeting and hear the family members talk about the kind of environment that would be best suited for patients with Alzheimer's disease. Weaver stresses, however, "in dealing with issues like these, the facilitator must be careful not to make the group members feel they are required to find a solution to a problem, but rather to create an environment where the members feel safe in discussing the issue."

Deborah Anderson has worked in mental health centers and has served as a professional facilitator. She has found that professional facilitators can be useful in the beginning by providing a "needs assessment" that can give the group a framework of issues. "Individual members can prepare a list of their needs. Then the best way to start a discussion is to deal with the most frequently listed needs first. Rigidly following the list, however, may not always be the right approach. Above all, the facilitator must be flexible and not follow a program for the sake of following a program."

Anderson also points out that "knowing what fails is as important as knowing what succeeds." To illustrate her point, she recounts the experience of an agency that developed a support group for Sudden Infant Death Syndrome. "The group met at the encouragement of an agency, and became a place where the parents could vent their feelings of loss and grief. But, since there was no positive step or constructive task that the leader or the members could accomplish, the group ultimately fell apart."

An important issue that is too frequently overlooked, says Anderson, is whether a support group will focus exclusively on Alzheimer's patients or will it include individuals with other forms of dementia as well. A group needs to determine if behavior will be the criterion for membership or if a group will consist of only those diagnosed as having Alzheimer's-type dementia. By using behavior as a criterion, groups could meet a broad array of needs. After all, it is not uncommon for individuals to be misdiagnosed.

Accurate diagnosis and assessment of patients are essential. There can be a great similarity in behaviors between the various types of dementias, but screening to eliminate non-organic problems is important for any disorder. Since a major function of support groups is dealing with the behavioral aspects of the disease, excluding individuals because they do not have a specific diagnosis of Alzheimer's disease may not be in the best interest of the group or the individuals the group is trying to serve. Flexibility in meeting these different needs is important, especially in the more rural areas where there is not a broad range of assessment and support services.

The importance of focusing cannot be ignored. Anderson has seen cases where support groups were established to meet the needs of adult children with aging parents, but the range of problems and the immediacy of concerns were often so different that the participants could not find many common elements. "Many groups can have the potential to be helpful, but if the groups try to cover too many areas they will not meet the needs of the members. Deciding what to focus on is critical, whether it is Alzheimer's caregivers or whether it is Alzheimer's disease and other dementias: there must be a common recognized goal that can be achieved." Anderson also stresses size as a factor in group development. While groups may vary in size from ten to twenty-five members, "anything larger than twenty-five tends to become a crowd. An ongoing group of that size makes constructive discussion difficult. If there are more than twenty-five people on a continuing basis, it would be best to divide into smaller groups so that everyone has a chance to be heard and participate."

Weaver recommends that education should not be the primary purpose of a support group. Information on legal, financial, and related issues must be generally addressed, the specific assistance with these issues can and must be obtained from other sources. Several meetings can focus on educational issues, but if education is the ultimate goal, the support group probably will not serve enough needs to keep it going.

Weaver recommends that groups just starting out develop a "mission statement," i.e., define purposes of the group and the goals it wants to accomplish. Another useful purpose of the mission statement besides helping the members clarify what they want from a support group, is to solve potential conflict between agency goals and individual interests. "Sometimes the sponsoring agency may have planned the support group with the purpose of developing a continuum of care for family caregivers. If an agency does develop such a continuum, they need to have resources in the community to support it. The members may not be looking that far ahead and simply see the support group as a place where they can address common problems. The two different purposes don't have to be mutually exclusive as long as the members are not made to feel that they are responsible for meeting the strict requirements of the agency."

Weaver also suggests that if there are a sufficient number of individual members with special interests, such as advocacy, they can form a separate public relations group. Different functions for different groups, will become more clear, Weaver suggests, if the mission statement is clearly outlined. The original mission statement, therefore, is an extremely important ingredient because it can shape the entire focus and direction of a group.

"The most essential ingredient for a successful group is the original planner," according to Weaver. "He or she must have an idea of the direction of the group. If a caring group is planned for, the support and acceptance it is designed to produce can happen. If a public relations group is planned for, it can happen. Groups get what they plan for, and therefore, they need a definition and they need good planning. A notice in the paper might be a way of finding people, but they will not stay in the group unless the members can define what they want and work together to get it."

As both Anderson and Weaver emphasized, groups started by a professional or an agency may be prone to confusion because of the sometimes differing purposes and goals of the agency and individual caregivers. Providers or agency personnel who assist in organizing support groups can be instrumental in framing the group's mission statement and assisting the members in defining their particular immediate needs.

Summary

These different experiences have demonstrated one essential feature: support groups must meet the needs of the caregivers. They must be places that provide emotional support, confidentiality, and an understanding of the caregiver's difficult role. The group must be a place not only where members can be educated about the disease, but also educate the caregiver in the necessity for self-care. They ultimately must be a place where the caregiver finds the strength and encouragement to continue. To be effective, they must provide a source of safety, comfort, solace, and endurance.

Some Practical Strategies for the Caregiver

Judy Gellatly, M.S.W.

The following is a partial list of practical ideas
for Alzheimer's caregivers. The list is abstracted
from materials I have developed over the years,
both as a caregiver and as a support group facilitator. It is offered here in the hope that it will
be useful to those in a daily caregiving situation.

I. Plan for the Possibilities

As someone undertakes the difficult role of caregiver for an Alzheimer's patient, there are many
issues to be faced and for which the caretaker
needs to be prepared. The following are some of
the more important items that need to be addressed:

♦ Learn everything you can about the disease.
Read books, articles, and case histories. Talk
with physicians and other caregivers. The more
informed you are, the better able you will be to
cope with the situation.

♦ Mobilize a group of people who can help you
when you need help: family, friends, physician,
psychiatrists, minister, priest, social worker,
nurse, therapist, counselor, lawyer, sitter, or
respite worker. Do not be afraid to ask for help
and advice.

♦ Decide which person in the group will serve
as the case manager, i.e., who will be the person
to help you evaluate the on-going status of your
patient and help you in making decisions about the
patient's functioning and the types of care he or
she needs. Involving someone else in the decision-
making process will enable you to make the best
possible decision.

♦ Obtain a durable power of attorney while your patient can still understand the procedure and can sign the power of attorney document.

♦ Plan a life for yourself in addition to the caregiving time. Take time away from your daily responsibilities and pursue your own interests. This will not only give you strength to go on, but will reinforce your self-esteem and enable you to see that there is life beyond caregiving.

♦ Monitor your own health. Have a complete check-up regularly. You will do both yourself and your patient harm if you do not care for your own health and keep up your strength.

♦ Find out about Alzheimer's disease support groups through the national organization, the Alzheimer's Disease and Related Disorders Association (ADRDA), or through its local chapter. If no group exists, contact your local Area Agency on Aging and see if a group exists.

♦ Make contact with other caregivers who are in similar situations.

II. Assess Your Patient

It is important to assess the ability of the person you are caring for to determine the level of function or dysfunction. One of the useful ways is to keep a written journal listing the patient's abilities and disabilities that focus on:

♦ speech: Assess the clarity of speech, the ease of word retrieval, the extent to which the patient stammers or repeats words and phrases;

♦ vision: Does the patient have difficulty reading; does he or she perceive color or have good distance vision? and so forth;

♦ memory: What kinds of memory does the patient have trouble with? Recent memories, long-term memories. What is the person's memory span if given instructions? Five minutes, ten minutes. Is the memory getting worse or remaining the same?

♦ orientation: Does the caree know where he or she is and with whom? Does he or she still have a comprehension of time, place, etc.

♦ anxiety: Some of the symptoms of anxiety include flushes in the face and neck, cold toes and fingers, rapid shallow breathing, sweaty palms, enlarged pupils, fearfulness, excessive irritability, and quick temper.

♦ depression: Is the patient persistently despairing and anxious?

By keeping a written record of these levels of functioning and dysfunctioning and checking on them periodically, the caregiver can gain a better understanding of the particular problems that the patient is facing and whether the patient's abilities are deteriorating at a moderate or rapid rate.

III. Consider the Patient

In addition to keeping a record of specific areas of function and dysfunction, try also to assess the skills of the patient in daily living:

♦ List the skills, such as dressing, eating, using the toilet or shower or bath, that the patient can still do without assistance.

♦ Encourage the patient's self-esteem by not over-helping, even if the results do not measure up to your standards, e.g., eating with fingers, but still feeding self, or wearing mismatched socks.

♦ Maximize the patient's functional effectiveness, freedom, and dignity. The caree should be allowed, to the limit of his or her cognitive ability, to participate in the care and to choose how the remaining years will be spent.

♦ Arrange for periodic biomedical exams that include both psychosocial and medical components in order to revise the care plan, if necessary.

IV. Stages of Assessment

There are six stages when the patient needs to be assessed in terms of a caregiving plan:

♦ prediagnosis: Write down what triggers your concern that there may be something different about the patient and how the caree acts that was substantially different from earlier behavior.

♦ during diagnosis: This is typically a stage of denial by both the caregiver and the patient. It is important that a record be kept during this period to assist in clarifying the situation for yourself and the patient.

♦ post-diagnosis: During this time of anger, guilt, and sadness, it is important to watch for changes in behavior and level of functioning. Some of the behaviors could be attributed to depression, and physicians can be consulted.

♦ coping: Even day-to-day coping with the situation needs to be evaluated from time to time so that circumstances can be altered to ease the caregiving process or change the environment to make more choices possible and life less cluttered.

♦ maturation: As both the patient and the caregiver begin to accept the losses that stem from the disease, they will begin to live one day at a time.   There is a particular need at this time to evaluate and assess the situation and arrange caregiving and life for the patient so that each can retain a feeling of self-worth.

♦ separation: Eventually the patient will no longer be mentally in the world of those who love and care for him or her. A new round of assessment needs to be done at this time, and some changes made when the patient can no longer communicate needs and wants.

V.   Assessment of the Caregiver

It is essential that the caregiver make a realistic inventory of his or her own capabilities.   This should include both physical and mental abilities to assist in becoming aware of your fitness to continue as a caregiver.   It is important to know what kind of outside help you need, not only in terms of maintaining the home, but also in having some respite time. Read up on caregiving skills with such books as The 36-Hour Day; Alzheimer's Disease; and Dementia (see list of suggested readings, p. 83).

VI. Assessment of Your Lifestyle

In addition to determining your own abilities, you need to consider the physical place where you live. It may be best to move into a smaller or different space. Change becomes increasingly difficult for the patient as the illness progresses. You will need to see that the house is secure and that the patient cannot just wander out. Can the furniture be less cumbersomely arranged? Should you try to live all on one level and move a bedroom to the main floor to avoid the need to run up and down stairs for both you and the patient.

Establishing a daily and weekly routine for your caree is important. Schedule activities such as dressing, eating, napping, bathing, and outings, and keep them to regular and anticipated times. Be certain to include in this, time for yourself.

Continue these assessments at intervals to accept and adapt to changes in your patient and your needs as a caregiver and as an individual. Stand back and look at your situation as changes need to be made, in relationships, in techniques, in arrangements. Include supportive family members and friends in these evaluations.

VII. Check Out Community Resources

There are many different types of resources in different communities. The best sources of information are Area Agencies on Aging and Senior Information and Referral lines in your local area. Libraries and service organizations can be of assistance also. You will need information on the following:

Daycare centers; senior centers; mental health centers; chore services; sitters; home nursing care; footcare; meals on wheels; respite services, and so forth.

VIII.   Communication Skills: Oral

Communicating with a patient with Alzheimer's disease is a difficult task. You can assist in the process by developing some communications skills. First, be certain that the patient does not suffer from hearing loss.

♦ Speak in a low, calm, slow manner.
♦ Make eye contact when speaking.
♦ Use short sentences.
♦ Always use the same word for the same thing.
♦ If giving instructions for a task, make sure the patient understands. If you are not understood, give assistance with gestures, or calmly repeat. Allow time for completion, as well as time for the patient to focus on the task before it is begun.
♦ Do not argue. Agree, then distract, divert, and then try again.
♦ Do not disagree with a fantastic statement by the patient.
♦ Agree, distract, and in a non-emotional manner divert into reality, very gently.

Index

Acetylcholine, 13, 14
Aging network, 86
Agnosia, 25
Alcoholism, chronic, 30, 32
Alzheimer's Disease and Related Disorders Association (ADRDA), 53, 74, 85, 93, 103
Alzheimer's Support, Information, and Service Team, 103
Aphasia, 10
Apraxia, 10, 25
Area Agency on Aging (AAA), 86
ASIST, 103
Assessment, 40, 68; multimodal, 40; initial interview, 40, 41, 43; screening instruments, 42; of onset, duration, and course of impairments, 43; ischemic score, 43; functional, 45, 46; Dementia Rating Scale, 47; memory and behavior checklist, 47; social and environmental, 48, 49; and support network, 50; laboratory tests, 50, 51; sensory and neurological, 51; neuropsychological,

51, 52; repeated testing for, 53; interpretation of tests, 53; and treatment, 58-60

Bereavement, 37; source of stress and depression, 36
Brain-cell abnormalities, 7

Caregiver, needs of, 67, 69, 70, 77-79
Caregiver support groups, 71, 81, 93; structure and activities of, 72, 74, 81; role of, 72, 74; leader's role in, 72, 75, 77, 96, 100, 103; goals of, 74; "rounds" of, 75; as social occasion, 78; and community resources, 80, 98; nursing home placement and, 80; and autopsy arrangements, 80; telephone network of, 81, 103; case histories, 95; formation of, 95, 97, 101; and families, 100; evolution of, 104; agency sponsored, 105; professional

facilitators and,
106, 107; and needs
assessment, 108;
mission statement,
109
Causation, theories
of, 18
Cerebral infarcts, 29
Cerebral lesions, 32
Choline, 15
Chronic brain syn-
drome, 4
Cognitive tests, 11
Cognitive impairment,
22; causes of 24,
50; reversible or
treatable sources
of, 31
Community resources,
85
Consciousness,
alteration in state
of, 25
Conservatorship,
88,90
Coping, 69
Creutzfeldt-Jacob
disease, 29
CT scan, 52

Delirium, 31
Dementia, 5, 37;
criteria for, 24;
multi-infarct, 29;
medication-related,
32; rating scales,
47, 54, 55, 57;
differential
diagnosis of, 52;
evaluation and
assessment of, 53,
54, 57; memory and

learning, 54; motor
and problem-solving
ability, 56
Dementias, non-
Alzheimer's, 7, 28
Denial, 68, 69
Depression, 32, 33,
36, 44, 45; Zung
Self-Rating Scale,
44; Hamilton Rating
Scale, 44, Beck
Inventory, 45;
Center for Epidem-
iologic Studies
Scale, 45;
Geriatric Scale, 45
Diagnosis, 68;
neuropathological,
12; biochemical, 12
Diagnostic and
Statistical Manual
of Mental Disorders
(DSM-III), 24, 26,
33, 44
Dopamine ("L-Dopa"),
14
Drugs: effects, 31,
37; reactions, 32,
37
Dysthymic disorder,
34
Durable power of
attorney, 88, 89

Family, 41, 84-94
passim; common
concerns of, 46;
and caregiver
support groups, 100
Finances, 87, 90

Contributors

Deborah Anderson, M.S.W.   Until 1985, Deborah Anderson managed the Older Adults Program for the Eastside Mental Health Center in Bellevue, WA, and in that capacity developed the support group described in this volume. More recently, she has been instrumental in developing comprehensive support and case management networks for use by the families of patients with Alzheimer's disease.

Judy Gellatly, M.S.W.   Judy Gellatly is the spouse of an Alzheimer's patient; a social worker who specializes in counseling Alzheimer caregivers; and a founding member, past president, and support group leader for the Puget Sound Chapter of the Alzheimer's Disease and Related Disorders Association (formerly the Alzheimer's Support Information and Service Team/ASIST).

Paula Gilbreath.   Paula Gilbreath provided in-home care for her Alzheimer husband until his death in 1982. She then served for three years as office manager for the Puget Sound Chapter of the Alzheimer's Disease and Related Disorders Association.

Laura S. Keller, Ph.C.   At the time she contributed to this volume, Laura Keller was a clinical psychology intern at the University of Washington.   She is currently a clinical psychology doctoral candidate at the University of Minnesota.

Thomas H. Lampe, M.D.   Dr. Lampe is a staff psychiatrist and physician for the Geriatric Research, Education, and Clinical Center at the American Lake Veterans Administration Medical Center in Tacoma, WA.   He also is an instructor in the Department of Psychiatry and Behavioral Sciences at the University of Washington.

Kathleen O'Connor, M.A. At the time this book was developed, Kathleen O'Connor served as administrator of the Pacific Northwest Long-Term Care Center at the University of Washington; as editor of its New Report, she developed a special review issue on Alzheimer's disease. She currently serves on the board of directors of the Alzheimer's Disease and Related Disorders Association of Puget Sound, and on the Executive Committee of the University of Washington's Alzheimer's Disease Research Center. She edits the Center's newsletter, Dimensions. Through O'Connor Community Relations and Communications, she specializes in health project planning and management, and writing in the health care field.

Joyce Prothero, Ph.D. At the time the present volume was developed, Dr. Prothero served as the director of Education, Training, and Publications for the Pacific Northwest Long-Term Care Center and as education director for the University of Washington's Institute on Aging. In these capacities, she developed a comprehensive continuing education program for the Center and Institute consisting of extension and independent study courses, summer workshops, and issue-oriented conferences. She continues as education director for the Institute on Aging and now also serves as deputy director for the Northwest Geriatric Education Center.

Betty Jane Schmidt. In 1972, Betty Jane Schmidt's husband was diagnosed as having Alzheimer's disease. She cared for him at home until 1980 when he was admitted to the Veteran's Administration nursing home facility in Tacoma, WA. Since 1970 she has been associated with an Alzheimer support group in Wenatchee, as one of the three co-founders and as the group's facilitator.